Deb Madonna

Dedicated to

my family,

Marcel

Andrew, Justine, John, Rebecca, Mark, Amanda,

and Teddy

and my friend,

Marg Moxnes

and my friend,

Jamie Jones

"God gave us memory

so that we might have roses in December."

—James Barrie

a stroke

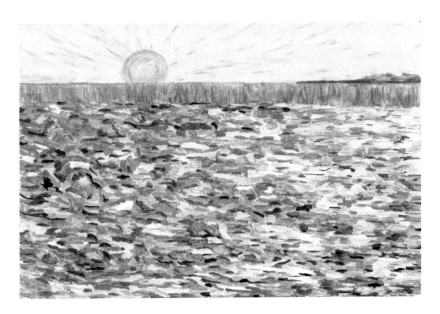

"Sunset"

one teeny, broken blood vessel

by Debra Madonna

CONTENTS

FOREWORD

by Justine Madonna

PRACTICALLY anyone with a personal phone is old enough to have received a phone call or text with sad news about a grandparent falling ill or passing on, or a friend in the hospital that has taken a turn for the worse. Receiving the phone call about Deb's stroke was nothing like those calls.

Deb wasn't the ill friend or family member. She wasn't the frail grandparent that there was some relief of pain. She is hard working, energetic, and busy with friends. She ate well and wasn't under the constant care of a physician; she wasn't jumping out of a plane, she wasn't a racecar driver, and she wasn't otherwise participating in other high risk activities. She was living a very normal day; we were all living a very normal day, not particularly worried about her activities and health at that moment. Things seemed "known", stable, and safe. Then, phone calls from our family started coming in and going out informing us that she had an aneurism: her brain was bleeding and might not stop.

The undercurrent of helplessness and frustration was consuming during the first few days. Our family dropped our silly, superficial activities and became laser focused on her condition, the data known and the unknowns, and hungry for more information immediately. Today, I am not confident that I accurately recall how long we monitored the bleeding in her brain; it feels like it had been over a week of agonizing waiting but it could have been two days or even just one. According to Deb's doctors that brain surgery was not an option; the MRI confirmed the bleed was in a place that could not be accessed with surgery. I wouldn't have thought I would be praying for brain surgery on a loved one until I had been told there wasn't anything the physicians could do. We would have to wait to see if her body repaired itself.

I cannot fathom how my father-in-law, Marcel, felt. He is her partner and she is his, in every sense I can imagine. His gaze toward her evidently carries love, respect, and support, but during this time, his face conveyed something that I don't have the courage to examine closely.

1

Next came the news that her brain *is* reabsorbing the blood. It was time to take a breath.

At my place of work that week, we had highly visible, highly strategic, and multi-day workshops with a regional and European team, and I held a unique and very necessary role in these sessions. Unfortunately, being in the room doesn't mean you're *in the room*. It had been a couple of days since Deb had been in the hospital, and at this point, we saw indication that her brain was absorbing the blood (i.e., brain surgery was no longer thought to be required), and she was conscious. My body was in one place while my head and heart were in Deb's hospital room. As my meetings were starting, we went around the room to "check-in" with each other and I noted to the group to please not be offended that day if they saw me checking my phone repeatedly as I was waiting on updates on my mother-in-law. My German colleagues assured me: "If you need to go, go. There is nothing more important." My co-workers extended a helping hand to me.

I left a few hours later and drove straight to Deb's hospital room and it was just the two of us. She doesn't remember this visit but I think I always will. She was calm, steady, and talking. Her experience in hospitals and helping others, I think, lends to her being very matter-of-fact about these things. I can still visualize her sitting in the bed, her legs out in front of her, wearing one of those terribly scratchy hospital gowns. I think what upsets me about her wearing the gown is that I know Deb shops with her hands, meaning, she touches every material before buying it and only dresses in things that feel good against her skin. This gown symbolized to me that none of this—Deb in this place and in this condition— made sense, as if there was some logic of right and wrong; she didn't deserve this.

We have to take the lead from Deb and not dwell on things that cannot be changed. She knew she needed to move forward and so shall we.

Deb is herself a clinician and that is what she asks from others for their assessments on her progress and manages expectations. In the long years of recovery, she has consistently been self-aware, communicating her progress openly with others, and she *has* been making progress. It has been over five years and she'll point out to others that a variation in the word she chose is part of her aphasia.

This is a woman who didn't accept an ongoing status-quo. She didn't see herself as a victim. She picked herself up while involving and pulling up those around her. Deb worked to achieve progress every day and her drive even increased drive when she learned she would be a grandma for the express purpose of giving her grandson the bonding experience with her as she had with her own grandparents.

For everyone learning about her journey, I hope this is a catalyst for growth in how to face challenges in your own lives. Deb chose to put her energy into understanding and tackling the path forward and bringing her loved ones along as partners. Effectively applying the finite energy we all have toward progress and recovery has resulted in her achieving her stretch goals. She rides her trike with her grandson; they play outside, on the floor, and go to the water park; they banter with each other, read, and do art projects. He has his Grammy at his side.

August 17, 2021

PREFACE

I make mistakes, always have, and always will. From the moment I was transported from a restaurant to the hospital, until today, the nature of those mistakes have changed, as well my comfort level with living with my mistakes, especially the little ones. Before I send a handwritten note or a typed message, I check and double check to make sure everything was correct: spelling, grammar and meaning. Now it takes effort to correct or even recognize or identify mistakes. In rehabilitation post stroke, every activity that therapists gave me was designed to restore function. The activities used in therapy were similar to what I did in kindergarten. I learned once and would have to learn again. Only this time, I had to patiently waiting for my brain to heal. Patience. Rest.

Some people are very particular and precise about what they say and write. Me, too. We each tolerate imperfections in others differently. You may be driven crazy by mistakes on the printed page. You may find there are misspellings, grammar errors on the pages in this story. As to why there is an error when there is spell check, I can explain, that due to aphasia, errors occur regularly in my writing and speaking. I am not proud if every word isn't perfect, but I am not ashamed or surprised. I was the school Spelling Bee champion in seventh grade, for heaven's sake. I did have help from editors and readers, extra sets of eyes, but the final thumbs up was mine. If there's an error anywhere in this story, circle them or dog-ear the pages, you may let me know and thank you. You may not want to read this part because it may sound like an excuse.

Aphasia: "loss or impairment of the power to use or comprehend words usually resulting from brain damage (as from a stroke, head injury, or infection)." (Merriam-Webster Dictionary)

I wanted to tell a story, and then finish the story, and put it between two covers, and set a copy on my bookshelf, and share it with others. My dilemma was finishing the story that may be imperfect or doing it now as is. I opted for NOW instead of perfect. I thought the story may have a value and an appeal to readers who aren't perfect either. When my son, John, was three years old, I said, "Please Hurry Up". John replied, "I am going as fast as I can". Yes, he was going as fast as he could. Aren't we all?

PART ONE

"A difference, to be a difference, must make a difference."

—Gertrude Stein

CHAPTER 1

A Mishap

The Brain's Stroke, (Cerebrovascular Accident, CVA)

IF anyone ever asks you if you would like to have a stroke, say, "No" or "No, thank you." The brain may warn you of an impending cerebrovascular accident, but the brain never asks permission. When I woke up in the Intensive Care Unit, (ICU), I opened my eyes for the first time in two days. My family was there, all together, in one room. I recognized them. That's what I remember of that day.

I experienced a CVA, a hemorrhagic stroke, ("a bleed"), on January 27, 2015, resulting in brain damage to a spot deep in my brain, the basal ganglia, thalamus. Despite this attack, my brain continued to repair herself from the moment the stroke began and it continues today. My brain made new neural pathways, compensating for losses: use of my right side, expressive speech, receptive taste, and in general, taking care of myself. I did not receive a written list of everything in my body that would be affected; I would discover that in time. My brain provided guidance. My body provided sweat and somewhere inside me, faith. I cooperated and I rested. Friends and family told me, "In six months, you will be your old self, good as new." Six months later, I was still trying to find my "old self". The "new me" was wobblier than the "old me". I will never be exactly like I used to be, which was not perfect to begin with.

This is the story about what I could not do that day when the CVA occurred, what I can do now, and what I still cannot do… yet. What happened to me affected my family. If there were different details, if I had had the stroke on a different day, or if a different spot in my brain had been damaged, it would be a different story. If I had a different family and different hospitals and medical helpers, that would have been a different story, too. I survived that stroke. I started over. I recovered. I thrived.

I wanted to understand everything that happened to me, everything about everything. My family and friends wanted me to be well. While I was in the hospital and the rehabilitation unit, my goal was to recover. My husband wanted me to regain the use of my right hand and to be able to walk on my own. When I went home, I was focused on what I needed to do, who was going to help me, and where I had to go to find help. Getting back to life required taking many baby steps.

Every Breath

IT was 1983. I had to leave my newborn son with a neighbor during the day for a few months while I completed an internship, an Occupational Therapy field placement, at St. Mary Mercy Hospital. I worked primarily with patients who had experienced cardiac events and strokes. "Every Breath You Take" was the song I listened to over and over in the car. I cried sad tears when I left my son, Andrew, with my very caring neighbor, Gayle Harshman, and her daughter, Kristen, on the way to work and happy tears when I picked Andrew up at the end of the day, and we went home.

1993 – 2014. I worked at St. Mary Mercy Hospital in the Marian Women's Center and the Behavior Medicine Unit.

On January 27, 2015, I entered St. Mary Mercy Hospital on a gurney, accompanied by Emergency Medical Technicians. I was not aware of anything happening to me. I was alone until someone contacted my family and let them know where I was. They quickly joined me.

On February 20, 2015, I left St. Mary Mercy Hospital, sitting up in a wheelchair and talking to my husband. My family joined us at our home.

I was familiar with the hospital. I had been a patient there on several occasions and an employee for 21 years. When I was an employee, I was respectful, helpful, and I provided the best care to those in the hospital. When I was a patient, I assumed that if I did that for others, then the caregivers in the hospital would do the same for me.

I wondered about other patients, especially the stroke patients. They may be frightened of hospitals and doctors. They may dislike the smells, colors, and all things normally found in hospitals. They were not comfortable around doctors or illness. It may be terrifying for them to wake up and realize they could not move a part of their body. They may not understand what was being said and worst of all, discovered that no one could understand them. Their families may feel the same way.

Flora and C.W.

WHEN I was a little girl, I followed my grandmother, Flora, everywhere. I was her shadow. That was how I got to know her. Flora worked very long hours, watching over our thirty-acre farm, in the greenhouse, planting and harvesting fruits, vegetables, taking care of chickens, goats and a baby calf every day of her life. I don't remember her sitting down unless it was a special occasion. She offered me fifty cents to weed the garden. I would last about ten minutes. She gave me fifty cents anyway and money to give to my brothers. Flora and C.W. would get up in the middle of the night to check on the plants in the greenhouse, to make sure there was a fire in the furnace in the winter, and water everything in the hottest part of the summer. Flora always noticed what I was wearing. She loved my soft, colorful clothes. I didn't realize that I loved them, too, until my friend, Gail Maloney, pointed out that I was like Flora when I was shopping for clothes. It may explain why I named one of my soft little kittens, "Flora." It may also explain why I know how to work hard.

During the last years of her life, Flora became confused. She wandered away from home. She was lost too often, but my grandfather, C.W., called one neighbor to tell him that Flora had wandered away. That neighbor called other neighbors. When they found her, they gently guided her home. One time Flora was discovered in a shallow hole. All curled up, she looked like a bird in a nest. Flora had frequent falls and she lost her ability to speak. Even with all her losses, she was still very sweet. For the last three years of her life, Flora was confined to bed, in a semi-conscious state, but she was at home and C.W. took care of her. Whenever I visited, C.W. and Flora, I would sit on one side of her bed and C.W., sitting across from me, telling me story after story about Flora and their life together. C.W. talked to her all the time, maybe more than he ever did before. After all their 64 years together, C.W. discovered that Flora had beautiful blue eyes.

Flora is always with me, but even more so these last few years, when I was confused, walking very clumsily, and fumbling for the right words. Even now she makes me less lonely. I am still following her shadow.

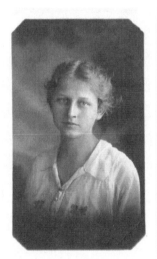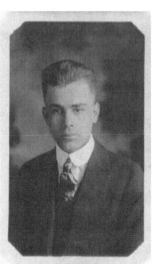

(Flora and C.W., Clarion)

CHAPTER 2

Postscript: A Broken Capillary vs. The Virus

April 29, 2020

When This Is Over

I began writing the story of the hemorrhagic stroke on January 27, 2020, the five-year mark post-stroke. That was my goal and I met it. I began editing and I was making progress. My intention was to write what I observed while I was in the hospital and at home. I wanted a record of the people, therapies, and activities that made a significant impact on my life.

That is what I had planned to do. And then, we found ourselves in the middle of a pandemic. I set my story aside. What relevance would a story about one person and one stroke have in a world fighting Covid-19? The ongoing coverage is overwhelming and we are unsure what comes next.

The story I had written had become ancient history in just a few weeks. I wrote about being saved, cared for, and helped back onto my feet. I wanted to acknowledge those who had helped, used what they knew, what I had needed, and the difference it made in my life. My experience was successful because the odds were in my favor, one person helped by dozens and dozens of people: first responders, medical personnel, family, and friends. I was never alone. Never. When I wrote, "If a different part of my brain had been damaged or if I lived in another city, it would be a different story. If I had had a different family and different helpers, that certainly would have been a different story, too". I did not know how different life would become.

Covid-19 and my stroke have one thing in common: the helpers. A stroke stopped me abruptly. The world continued on and, when possible, I rejoined the world around me. Covid-19 stopped the world abruptly. The microscopic Covid-19 has powers we cannot ignore. The world turned upside down and the odds are not in favor of patients, their families, the healthcare community, and first responders. It is terrifying for the caregivers to do their job when they are outnumbered and do not have the tools they need.

The first responders, nurses, and doctors are front and center, working under extraordinary conditions because they are extraordinary. They do everything they were trained to do under conditions in which no one should have to work. Even though the number of people contracting, becoming ill, and / or dying from Covid-19 has been is staggering. Medical teams continue fighting for every human being in their care. Medical personnel stay with a patient because families are not allowed to be with the patient. First responders and medical personnel do not run away from patients even when their lives are in danger. Through the Covid-19 months, we heard the medical people speaking strongly to let us know that we all need to think of others and to work together.

Here we are in 2020 and our list of helpers is growing because they are needed. In addition to first responders and medical teams, there are now grocery store workers, housekeepers, janitors, sanitation engineers, teachers who are teaching their students, delivery people, and all who work so the rest of us can stay home and be safe. They are all essential workers now. When I was in the hospital, my helpers sent me cards and flowers and drove me to doctor appointments. The 2020 helpers today are making masks.

On April 16, 2020, the Mayor of Livonia, Maureen Brosnan, joined firefighters, police, rescue workers from Livonia and other communities as they drove up to St. Mary Mercy Hospital. ("At St. Mary Mercy in Livonia where hospital staff are receiving thanks from police and fire", *Hometown Life / Livonia Observer, April 16, 2020*). If you know a healthcare worker, ask them why they do what they do.

Several years ago, I was a member of a committee who awards vocational scholarships to high school seniors who were pursuing a trade or skill after graduation. Listening to young people share their goals and dreams made me hopeful and proud. One of the young men stated that he wanted to be a firefighter. One of the committee members asked the young man why he wanted to be a firefighter, and he answered, "I want to save people". Asked that question, another person may give a very long answer. This young man wanted to save people. No doubts. Our country is blessed to have so many people who want to take care of people and save people. That was a great afternoon. He received a scholarship.

Fred Rogers said to look for helpers when times are tough. The helpers demonstrate their faith by staying by our side. When this is all over, someone will write an anthem for the helpers.

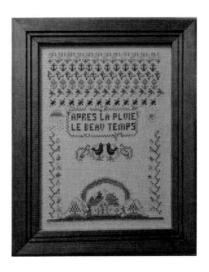

(This sampler was made by my friend, Marg Moxnes, many years ago. "Après La Pluie Le Beau Temps". "After the rain, the good times.")

Thoughts

The words are
"Thank you".
Now is the time to say them.

I didn't know
if I would see you again,
but here you are
and here I am.

It is amazing how little things have the power to lift my spirit.
I almost forgot how to play,
but you reminded me.
Thank you.

John said you called;
He wrote your message on a pink index card.
"Everything is fine.
See you on Sunday."

sigh and thank you!

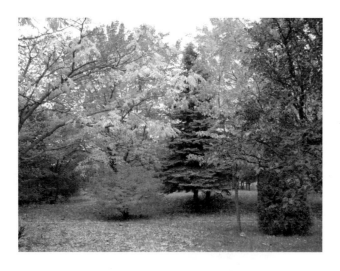

PART TWO

I am optimistic,
       but I am not an optimist.
I am a poet.

CHAPTER 3

CHANGE OF PLANS

Ladies Who Lunch

Thank goodness for facebook reminders:

1.26.15. 6:02 a.m.

Cindy: "Dress warm, stay safe, have a great day!!! Looking forward to my luncheon with my dear cousin, Deb"

Trisha: "When are you going?"

HAVING lunch with my cousins, Cindy Davis Peters and Trisha Peters, is always a treat, even though it doesn't happen very often. When we meet, the first thing we say is how silly it is that it has taken so long to get together. I do not remember what we had for lunch, but we were happy. We talked and laughed. The food was delicious. Throughout lunch, though, I was missing some of the words of the conversation, fading in and out for a few seconds. I was struggling to stay in my chair. We made plans to see each other soon, hugged each other, and said goodbye. After lunch, I took care of a few items on my "to do" list.

1.27.15

Early Morning at Panera Bread

At Any Given Time, You May Be on Either End of a Helping Hand.

I drove to an early morning meeting. I was talking to people and answering my phone. Suddenly everything was quiet. My left hand was reaching across to my right side to hold on to something, anything. Someone asked me, "Are you okay?"

I answered "Sleepy" once or twice, and then my answer was, "No," and then I was unable to answer or hear anyone ask me anything.

Someone called 911. The EMTs transported a 63-year-old woman to the hospital. That was me. I do not remember anything else in the restaurant. I woke for a minute in the Emergency Room. An EMT walked by my room. That was all I remembered. I do not know how the EMTs knew who I was. I do not know how the people at the hospital knew who I was. I do not know who found my car. I do not know how my family found out I was in the hospital or what they were told. The next 48 hours were lost. I did not think about any of this for a few years. I probably should ask my family these questions and many more.

It was very cold the morning of 1.27.15. I wore my moose coat, with the moose buttons. It is green, woolen, ankle length, and very warm. I bought the coat at Zehnder's of Frankenmuth on an Annual Cousin's Day outing with my cousins Charlotte, Arline, Sandy, Marilyn, Carolyn, and Judy. I am not sure if this was the year Ginny and Jody were with us. I am so happy that my coat did not get lost in the chaos. I really love that coat.

1.27.15 – 1.28.15

4.6 x 2.2 x 3.2 cm

UPON my arrival at St. Mary Mercy Hospital, a Computerized Axial Tomography Scan (CAT scan) was taken. The scan indicated a cerebrovascular accident (CVA) had occurred, a hemorrhagic stroke. A capillary had burst in the left side of my brain, in the basal ganglia, resulting in a 4.6 x 2.2 x 3.2 cm hematoma. Surgery could not be performed because the bleed was too deep in my brain. My husband was told by doctors that there may be clinical deterioration and I may not be able to swallow, in which event, the recommendation would be that nasogastric tube feeding would be necessary. I was moved to the Intensive Care Unit (ICU). The bleed continued for two days. I survived only because a little capillary stopped bleeding by itself.

The first moments I was awake, I was aware: my family was in the room with me. There was no noise and no one was moving; my right leg and my arm were heavy and I was unable to move it. That is what I remembered of the day I woke up.

1.28.15 – 1.31.15

Repairs

AFTER a few days, I was moved from ICU to a Medical Floor and then to the In-Patient Rehabilitation (Rehab) Floor. It was now up to the Medical and Rehabilitation (Rehab) teams, aka Repair Crews, to keep me going forward. My family's role was to stand by. My job was to do whatever was prescribed. The Medical and Rehab teams set out to find what still worked, what could be fixed, mended, restored, and what had no hope of any of these.

If there is an interruption in the electrical system of my house, I can test the lights, the electrical appliances, the outlets. If all else fails, I can rip out all the dry wall to get to the wires. If I do not get all the lights to work, I can get a flashlight. There are instructions I can read to get the lights working again. Not so for my brain. Does it matter what spot in the brain is affected? Yes. It makes all the difference. The area affected determines what happens next in your life.

A human being's nervous system is more delicate and more complicated than the wiring in my house. A brain cannot be removed and inspected so one can figure out how to fix it. Amazingly, however, the human brain can rewire itself. Not the old way, but she may find a new route. In my case, I went along for the ride to see what I was able to do. Did I have a serious stroke? Yes, all strokes are serious, medically, and emotionally, for families too. While I was in the hospital, there was not a lot of laughter for my family. As for me, I was somewhere else. I was a little lost. I was so happy that I was staying in the hospital for rehabilitation. I asked Marcel over and over to find out if I was staying in the hospital for rehab. When he found out that I was staying, I was relieved. Keeping me in the hospital meant the medical staff thought I would make progress.1.29.15

Impact

THE impact of a stroke can be subtle or severe. In my case, the preliminary impact caused a severe interruption in my ability to function:

- Right-side hemiparesis (RS), weakness on right side of my body.
- Right-side abnormal body posture.
- Right central facial nerve weakness.
- Right-side neglect, both visually and sensory.
- Right arm was weaker than right leg. Right-side strength improved minimally over first few days.

- Babinski reflex on the right side, an abnormal reaction due to brain damage.

- Expressive Aphasia and Receptive Aphasia: a decreased ability to understand or express speech. There were some minor improvement over the first few days and progress continues to today.

- Dysarthria, slurred speech.

- Essential Hypertension, no known cause.

- Ability to swallow may be impaired, to be determined.

- Memory functions; to be determined.

Right-Side Hemiparesis (RS)

In a Cardiovascular Accident, (CVA), an injury on the left side of the brain affects the right side of the body, completely or partially. When I woke up in the ICU, I was unable to feel or move my right side. Then there was a flicker of movement at first. It would take days for any feeling to return. Function would return a little at a time. All the things that I could not do at first became the list of all the skills that I worked on with my family, therapists, nurses, and doctors:

- moving my right arm and leg

- moving in bed

- lifting my arms and legs

- sitting up in bed

- getting into a wheelchair

- getting to the bathroom

- eating with my left hand until I could use my right hand

- using my right hand for anything

- using a wheelchair, a walker, then a cane, and then holding onto to the arm of a helper until I could walk by myself

A top priority, from morning until night, was my safety. My right side had to be protected from, well, from me. I had to accept help and pay attention because I could get hurt. Keeping my helpers safe at all times was another priority. I would not intentionally hurt my right side, but I did not feel my right leg and arm. If I was not looking at my right side, I would forget it was there. I followed my helpers' instructions as my right side was not aware of its surroundings and its abilities. I developed strategies dependent on the increased sensations on my right side. At first I was not aware of anything around me. I could breathe on my own. Even making eye contact took time. In fact, everything took time and focused effort. Focus was a rare commodity for months. During the first week in the hospital, I didn't even look around me, but I could respond to what a person said, their voice and face. I could focus on one person at a time.

Starting in the second week, I didn't notice anything in cafeteria, except the food put in front of me. I wasn't hungry and food had no taste. When I returned to my room after the cafeteria and therapies, my room became more familiar because it was full of cards, presents and flowers, lots of flowers. Once that happened and I was a little more alert, then I could be more responsive during therapies.

What helped me the most was that I listened to everyone and I was willing to do whatever I was asked to do. I was never asked to be perfect. Years ago, I took a Brain Gym Class, Lucy French was the teacher. I may be doubtful about my ability to run a marathon, but I learned to say, "I can't run in a marathon … YET. That "yet" has been a lifesaver many times. I used "yet" many times each day in the hospital.

Sound simple? No, it was not simple. My balance was affected. When I sat, I leaned toward the right. I had to be positioned to avoid falls. If I was sitting in a wheelchair, my arm or leg could slip off the armrest or footrest into a wheel. Even laying in bed, my arm or leg could get caught in the bedrails and I would not know it. The only solution was that the staff and family had to be vigilant because I was not responsible. Blankets and pillows were used to position my body and protect my hand, arm, foot, and leg when I was in the wheelchair, sitting in a chair, or sitting on the therapy tables, and when I was in bed. Even though I did not feel my right arm or right leg, even though I could not move my right arm or right leg during the first week, I could feel caring, concern, hugs, and kisses from family and friends and staff.

Severe Expressive Aphasia

COMMUNICATION with others was challenging because I had to search for the right words to express myself and I had difficulty speaking in complete sentences. I was not aware that my speech was unclear when I regained consciousness after the stroke. I had a lot to say and I said it, even if I did not use the right words. My wrong words were related or they sounded similar. I intended to say, "I'm going to the dining room," but I said, "I am going to the movies." Others experience aphasia where the words have nothing in common. It is difficult to know if the person is thinking clearly and just having difficulty retrieving words. It can be a trying time for all. The words I used were not always correct. The right words were elusive. Aphasia worsened with frustration. The listener can keep the situation calm by listening with kindness, love, and more kindness, the best medicine for everyone.

Aphasia is still part of my life, in speech, listening, reading, and writing. It is rare that I can type a note without errors, even after reading and re-reading. It may take a day or two to get all the words correct, maybe. My hands have feelings do not "care" and do not get embarrassed when they send a text with typos or grammatical errors. My hands are trying. My brain is trying. I have improved over the last five years. I still continue to improve. Typing a letter, mixing aphasia with AutoCorrect, is like a roller coaster ride. It is exhausting. I just always blame AutoCorrect. I do not fret. I continue to use new skills and techniques to recover words and use them effortlessly.

One technique I use when I am typing a note is to include pictures in place of words. It helps to convey what I am thinking because I leave out a lot of words. It is awkward to answer a question or have a conversation. All the words I have ever known are still inside me. I have to reach up and grab those pesky words. Speech Therapy was invaluable for dealing with aphasia. I continue to do brain exercises, such as Brain Gym, a program used for movement and connecting my body with my thoughts. My strategies in dealing with aphasia:

Silence. Stop talking. Take a breath. Visualize what I intend to say. Take time. Rest.

- When I go to bed, I have a pad of paper and pencil on the nightstand. If I think of something, I write it down.

- If I am having a conversation and I cannot think of a word, it may come to me when I go to bed. I will send a text to the person I was talking to: "Darn it, Casablanca, Humphrey Bogart and Ingrid Bergman, of course."

- The "friends" technique: If you have friends who understand your aphasia, they can correct you. They may understand what you are trying to say and let it go. Give your friends permission to correct you when there are other people around.

- If I misspeak, please ask me if you do not understand what I said. For me, there will be no offense taken.

- Do not be embarrassed. If you are one of those people that hate getting notes with all those mistakes or thinks I am uneducated and I have A-P-H-A-S-I-A.

- Not all communication uses words. Kindness is more powerful than words. The medical staff was helpful and patient when I only had a few words. My family and friends were supportive when my speech was garbled. I knew when someone was angry, frustrated, or happy when not a word was not spoken.

- Whenever you spend time with good friends, everyone is laughing so hard, and you are having a hilarious time. Chances are no one is finishing a sentence. That is not aphasia.

- Yes, I have called my children by each other's name and sometimes by our pets' names. This is not aphasia; this is being a mom. I may not always use their correct name, but I know who they are. To any mom who does this, bless your heart, honey.

Severe Receptive Aphasia

DURING the first week in the hospital, I did not understand much that was going on. Everyone took care of me. The medical staff used simple instructions and I am sure they repeated what I needed to know as often as needed. My loving friends sent me so many flowers and 'Get Well' cards that they filled my hospital room. For several weeks, I could not read the words on a card or the name of the person who sent the flowers. When someone read the name to me, I knew exactly who the sender was. That's what I remember.

I still have difficulty with written and oral instructions and if someone tells me their phone number: "XXX-1234," I write down: "XXX-5678."

When I was home, I made a hair appointment for a Thursday at 11 a.m. I wrote the day, date, and time on a piece of paper and I read it back to Jenny Wendel, my hairdresser. I added it to my calendar. On Thursday, I checked my calendar and I had posted the appointment for 12 p.m. I called Jenny to confirm my appointment. It was 11 a.m. I didn't want to show up at the wrong time for a hair appointment with Jenny. Jenny has been my hairdresser and friend for thirty years. She did not have any children when I met her. Now she has three grown adult children and three grandchildren. We have commiserated, groaned, talked, chuckled, given updates about our children and grandchildren. I don't think we spent more than two or three minutes discussing hair styles. So you can see I have too much respect for Jenny than to be late for an appointment.

Aphasia: the Language with a Thousand Dialects

WHAT is your first language? English, French, Mandarin, Italian? No, our first language is the Human Language. This is how we communicate with the world before we use or understand words. A baby's language is smiles, giggles, different types of cries, crawling, reaching for items. A baby's reward is receiving smiles, food, or hugs. Spoken words have limited value; it's the tone, touch, and eye contact that tell the story. Babies will graduate from babble and gibberish to their first words. Babies learn to use words, not by guessing, but experimenting. The child's skills will continue till the end of her life or illness or injury that interferes with language. Adults may lose spoken language one day and they may return to babbling.

The loss for the adult and those around her may create turmoil. The adult who has a loss of right words will still attempt to be understood unless there is no one to hear. The adult's loss of language may be received with love or rejected with anger and frustration from the listener. A stroke took parts of my language, but not my spirit. I can assure you that I am thankful to the listener who will listen as if they have all the time in the world. To all listeners, please remember you are not the doctor, you are a human being. Your gift is your willingness to sit by someone's side. Do you have a pet? An animal can't talk and they may not understand your words either, but they'll stay by your side. We may not understand what an animal is trying to tell us, but they are forgiving. Spending time together makes our pets happy. That's all. How would Timmy have gotten out of the well? Lassie didn't just run home looking for help. Lassie made sure everyone understood that Timmy was in the well for heaven's sake. Lassie had a great gift which was good because Timmy often needed assistance.

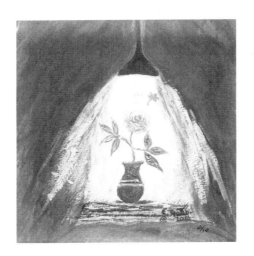

(Permission to use granted by artist, Ed Good)

Thoughts

I broke into a gazillion pieces, quietly, easily,
standing,
doing nothing in particular,
dawdling, lollygagging,
strolling,
not thinking of anything in particular.

Then,
a tumble turned into
a trip, a skid, a spill,
a plunge,
a free-falling crash,
landing, right there
at the place I needed to be,
broken into a gazillion pieces,
laying in a field of dandelions,
not far from the crossing of old self and new self.

someone picked me up.
he paused,
waited for the next train,
which was going to a very quiet
and peaceful place.
how did I know when I was home,
even fallen and broken?

I knew
because my family made a stunning kaleidoscope
out of the broken bits
to welcome me home.
they thought I would love it.
I did.
there is nothing more pleasant

than looking through a kaleidoscope,
finding sunshine and a bright blue sky

no matter how far away I have gone,
I always manage to get home,
where I belong.

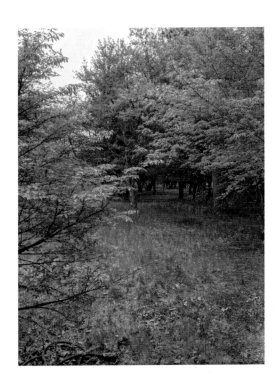

CHAPTER 4

How Long? Why? How Long?

Good Fortune

I was fortunate to live in a town where someone knew when to call 911, and the EMTs responded promptly, and that I was transported to a local hospital that was clean and safe. I was fortunate that the hospital personnel knew what to do to care for me as soon as the ambulance arrived at the hospital. I was evaluated, monitored, and treated. I was fortunate that the hospital personnel had a plan to move me from the Emergency Room, to a CAT Scan Room, to ICU, to a Medical Floor, to Rehab, (In-Patient Rehabilitation Unit), and finally, discharge me to my home.

Every staff person who came into my room confirmed that I was the patient they were supposed to see. They asked questions, wrote in a chart, and put the data in a computer so any one in the hospital could access my records when needed. I am not complaining, but my husband and sons were the ones who answered questions because I couldn't. Despite all the people who came in and out of my bubble, I rested. It was very quiet the first two days. I do not know who told the doctors I had a headache for the previous two days before the stroke occurred, but I do not remember having a headache. I did have facial droopiness, but I was fortunate that it soon went away.

In no particular order of importance, this is a partial list of the helpers: EMTs, Firemen, Policemen, Emergency Room, Attending Doctors, Nurses, Lab Technicians, Radiologists, Neurologists, Neurosurgeons, Physical Medicine Doctors, Cardiologists, Residents, Housekeepers, Attending Physicians, Consulting Physicians, Sonographers, Admitting Physicians, Rehabilitation Doctors, Occupational Therapists, Physical Therapists, Speech Therapists, Social Workers, Chaplains, Aides, Dieticians, Dining Room staff, and more. I am sure I have left someone off this list.

Every one of these people did at least one thing that was part of my initial care and recovery. You may not like everyone who came into your space, but they had a skill that I benefited from. Geez, I was not going to marry them, for heaven's sake! Fortunately, the people I met were kind and considerate. I needed help with everything, starting with surviving the stroke and dozens of other things. All these people were human beings doing their job the best they could for someone they did not know. I did know one of the rescue team who arrived at the coffee shop, who assessed what I needed, and lifted me into the ambulance; he will always be my hero. To all the human beings that helped me, thank you for helping me to get to where I am today. I wanted you know that I noticed.

Tip: My grandfathers taught me something very important: Be pleasant, especially when you are in the hospital. No matter how poorly you feel, be very polite and cooperative. Do not be mean. If you are nasty, you will not get any Tapioca or help going to the bathroom. If you are feeling horrible, try not to be ornery all the time. It won't make you feel better.

How Long?

"HOW long" is a million-dollar question? "How long" will I be in the hospital? "How long" before I can walk by myself? "How long" until I can cut up my own food? "How long" until I can drive? "How long?" "How long?" "How long?" The answer is, "It will take as long as it takes." A better question is, "What can I expect tomorrow? Okay."

Good People

SO why did I have a stroke? There was either a flaw in a capillary deep in my brain and my blood pressure may have been a little too high. The end result was a burst blood vessel filling my brain with fluid, my own blood. I eat healthy foods, plenty of fruits and vegetables. I stay away from things that I should stay away from, such as salt, foods high in salt, and aggravation. Aggravation may not have a negative effect on everyone, but it is not good for me. I exercise as I am able and I had never been diagnosed with high blood pressure. I take care of myself which has been invaluable during recovery and rehabilitation. It did not prevent the stroke that I had, but it may have prevented a more extensive incident.

Some people are surprised when someone they know has an illness or accident. Their reaction may be, "Why do bad things happen to good people?" I learned that being a good person does not prevent a stroke. Why me? Why did I have a stroke? Because I did.

Causes

"READ the Fine Print." Strokes can be treated and prevented. People have been known to miss or ignore the warning signs. Do not be the person who ignores warning signs and does not ever "Read the Fine Print." The causes that led up to my stroke may have been building for a long time. A stroke is either the sudden blockage of arteries, which is called an ischemic stroke, or a ruptured blood vessel in the brain to bleed and to pool, which is called a hemorrhagic stroke. There are medications that may be able to break up a clot (ischemic). If there is a bleed (hemorrhagic), surgery may be performed. In my case, surgery was not possible because the location of the bleed was deep inside my brain. If the blood flow to an area of the brain is deprived of oxygen for 3 or 4 minutes, can damage or kill brain cells can be life threatening. During recovery, the rest of the brain continues operating, while attempting to make new connections to compensate for the damaged area.

I refer to "my stroke" because it damaged my brain. I could also call it "our stroke" because it affected my family, too.

Risk Factors

I know, I know, I know. "Do This and Do Not Do That." No one likes to be told what to do. It is your decision, but I would suggest that you consider having a yearly physical. Monitor your blood pressure. A measurement of 120/80 mm is considered to be the normal range. Assess your overall health. This is important to know. Take care of yourself every day.

My Risk Factors

- 63 years old
- undiagnosed high blood pressure
- possibly a weak spot in a blood vessel, unknown
- family history of strokes or heart attacks

There may have been other factors. Over time, I discovered that salt and stress had a negative impact on my blood pressure. I never knew what high blood pressure felt like. After the stroke, occasionally my blood pressure was elevated. I had felt the pressure, not pain, in my brain, in reaction from agitation and salty foods. There was a feeling sometimes that "I could not think". Do not play with stress; do not underestimate the damage that stress can have on you. Be aware of unnecessary stressors that affect you, physical and emotional. We all recognize how a car accident is a stressor, but don't dismiss the little stressors that happen every day. Would you believe that some people get upset about someone leaving shoes in the front entryway as when someone is ill? Some people become upset when another person loads the dishwasher the "wrong" way. And if anyone points out that there is not a "right" way to load the dishwasher. Watch out. We humans may pump out the same amount of adrenaline when there is an argument over the dishwasher, hissy fits, tantrums, and a tornado. Watch out for hissy fits and tantrums whatever the reason. At one time, I have to admit that I would become a little irritated when no one emptied the clean dishes out of the dishwasher or put the dirty dishes into the dishwasher.

Several months after the initial stroke, I had a second CT scan to determine if there were any other suspicious areas to be concerned about; nothing was observed. I take medication for high blood pressure, which has been effective. I monitor my blood pressure once a day, limit my salt intake, drink six to eight cups of water daily, and get plenty of sleep (6–8 hours).

Other Risk Factors (that do not apply to me *now*)

- overuse of blood thinners

- physical inactivity

- heavy drinking

- use of illicit drugs, such as cocaine and methamphetamine

- cigarette smoking

- high cholesterol

- diabetes

- heart disease

- hormones

- atrial fibrillation

- etc., etc., etc.

January 29, 2015
Three Days Post Stroke (PS)

Lovely Phone Calls, Texts, and Flowers

NOTES, cards, gifts, emails, texts, facebook posts, visitors, and oh so many flowers arrived throughout the day and evening of day three post-stroke. I became aware of incoming messages on day four or five. My family read all the messages to me because I could not, but I knew who they were talking about. I saved everything so I could read all of them when I got home. I felt everyone was pulling for me and so thankful for their thoughtfulness. Caring gestures are powerful medicine. It is true; look it up. It was a bridge between friends and friendships, new, old and forever. The hospital staff dropped into my room to see the daily deliveries. The flowers and cards and gifts made me a real person, not just the "Patient in Room 222." You can never have enough flowers, cards or friends.

When I had been in the hospital a week, my friend, Gail Maloney, whispered in Marcel's ear, "When Deb gets through this; take her to Paris, for heaven's sake."

Week One
Intensive Care Unit (ICU), Medical Floor, Rehabilitation Unit (Rehab)

Make a Good Impression

WITHOUT jumping too far ahead, I rested, rested, rested, so that at the end of the week I could be moved to the rehab floor. I was very anxious about moving to rehab. I was not nervous, but I knew that if the medical team decided I was stable and that I would make progress, I would be moved from the medical floor to the hospital's In-Patient Rehabilitation Floor (I-P Rehab). If they felt I was unable to progress, they may send me to an outside rehab facility. That may not be true, but that is what I thought. I wanted to rehab in this hospital.

Sunday, February 1, 2015
Last Day of Week One

Moving from the Medical floor to the Hospital's Inpatient Rehabilitation Floor

I would have checked for monsters under my bed, but I can't because I can't get out of bed by myself. I will ask my husband to look.

Hurray! I was moved to the Rehab Unit in the Hospital about 9 p.m., Sunday evening. I was a patient in the hospital that I worked in for 21 years. I had been on my best behavior because I wanted to stay there for my recovery. Everything was familiar, I understood the routine and I was relieved. Marcel, my husband, and Mark, my son, gathered all my belongings, cards, presents, and flowers—and took them to my new room. They stayed as I got settled for the rest of the night.

The medical staff was wonderful and helpful, with the exception of one. On the first night on the rehab unit, a nurse who had my room assignment really upset me. In the morning, I told my husband about the nurse. When the head nurse of the unit stopped in to see me in the morning, I told her, too. I doubt that I explained clearly what bothered me, but they understood that I was upset. The head nurse apologized and promised that the nurse would not be assigned to me again. It is always important to speak up for yourself.

It was my first night in the rehab unit on the midnight shift. I was still unable to get up by myself. After ringing the buzzer the third or fourth time, she was irritated with me, my impression. In the middle of the night, in a new place, and I was all by myself, I was unable to clearly say what I needed. I handled the situation the best I could. I put the blanket over my head and stayed there all night. I can say that the nurse had not done anything horrible, but I don't often usually pull a blanket over my head because I am afraid. I do not know if I could have spoken up if I had not worked at the hospital and had a supportive family. It was important to clarify what had happened. so this one experience did not cloud my impressions of everyone else I encountered. What I know for sure that nurse did not come to work that night to make a patient afraid.

It was helpful to be surrounded by people who jumped in whenever needed and to be my voice. As it got later on the second night, I became very apprehensive. Starting that night Marcel and my friends, Gail Maloney and Ruth Martin, took turns magically appearing at 9 p.m. and curling up in the very uncomfortable chair next to my bed until morning. My apprehension disappeared. I do not know what my nights would have been without my nighttime posse. After dinner each night, the nurses asked me who was staying with me that night.

Monday, February 2, 2015
Week Two, First Morning
Rehabilitation (Rehab)

Recovery, Rehabilitation, Resting, and Healing

WHEN you have a stroke, even in a small, spot, the whole brain has to rest, sometimes for a long time. Rest

For the first week of my hospitalization, I was not asked to do anything. Starting bright and early on the first morning of week two, first day of rehab, an aide helped me wash, dress, and get into the wheelchair. She transported me to the dining room for breakfast where I sat at a table all by myself; I was a little lost. The staff brought me breakfast and checked with me to see if there was anything I needed; I did not know what I needed.

No one pointed out that I was a little sloppy. That was to be expected; we both knew that. Aides shuttled me to an hour of Occupational Therapy, an hour of Physical Therapy, two 30-minute sessions of Speech Therapy, my room, lunch, and dinner. Later in the evening, an aide helped me change from my street clothes to pajamas. The medical staff checked on me throughout the day.

At the end of the first day on the rehab unit, I learned how little I could do for myself. I was not allowed to move around the room or the rehab unit by myself, not even from the bed to a chair. I could move around my room the last week I was in the hospital, but nowhere else. I never said, "I feel terrible because people have to help me." Boo hoo. I didn't say it because it made me sound foolish. The help was there because I needed it and it would be there as long as I needed it. I was weak. I had difficulty following directions. I could not even take baby steps by myself, not even very little bitty steps. My husband said I was doing a little better every day. He was right.

Fatigue

I was tired when I sat up in bed, visited with family, and when I laid in bed. I was tired when I had visitors and when someone read my cards and notes. The therapies really wore me out. I was fatigued, not just a little sleepy, but so tired I could not think. The fatigue meant my brain was recovering. I cooperated and took a lot of naps. I never complained because I am a great napper. I napped and still slept all night.

Cold

I was always cold. For the longest time, I was the one who was chilly, wore a sweater and covered with a blanket or two. Even going through menopause, no matter how big the hot flash was, I was cold. While I was in the hospital, I needed blankets, more blankets and my new quilt from my friend, Ruth Martin. It would be several years before I was warm again. Over the last year, I am not cold. In fact, even when it is cool outside, I am comfortable. It's a little thing, but significant to me.

I Owe Somebody A Lot of Money

NO matter what you think should be done about our system of health care, we have to figure out what we want, how to pay for it, and available to all. Stop arguing. It is really easy to think we can cut back, but where? I had a brain bleed resulting in a 4.6 x 2.2 x 3.2 cm hematoma within the left lentiform nucleus of the basal ganglia. The bleed stopped on its own after two days, but it has taken years to recover. What is the cost of fixing me with insurance and without?

Where should we cut? Maybe we cut 911 or the First Responders that came to the restaurant, treated me, and transported me to the hospital. Maybe someone should have told the manager of the restaurant to prop me in a corner until my family could pick me up and take me home. Once I was home, hope for the best.

Imagine what it would have been like five years ago, ten years, or fifty years ago. Imagine the remarkable advances and more to come that we do not know about yet. It is something to be proud of. We should insist that this is the standard. How can we have what is needed to take care of people and not use it?

In the 1940s, my grandmother, Flora, had a car accident. The car hit a pothole. There were no seatbelts or airbags. Her right leg was shattered. There was no reconstructive surgery, just pins. She stayed in the hospital for six weeks. She remained in bed while in the hospital. She did not receive therapies. Visiting hours were limited, as well as who could visit. Her right leg was three inches shorter than her left leg. She never received orthotics for her shoe. There were no programs to aid her in her recovery, except the "Good Luck to You" program. Flora was left to heal on her own. The accident changed her life negatively and dramatically. I can just imagine how much pain she must have been in, while in the hospital, and for the rest of her life. Flora must have been scared and lonely.

The health care that I received does exist. I am proof that everything I needed, I received. The question is why it isn't available for all. I do believe that I would have avoided having a stroke if I was aware that my blood pressure had been discovered and treated. If I had taken my blood pressure at home once a day and not just at an annual physical, it may have been helpful. I have a twenty dollar high blood pressure cuff and I monitor my pressure once a day. I take blood pressure medication which is fairly inexpensive. So, do we find solutions to provide the best health care to everyone or not? We are pretty smart, but wishing for the best is not a viable solution. A spoonful of sugar does not make everything feel better.

Thoughts

A Quiet Crash

It is true
that when some people experience a stroke,
they may feel a dull ache,
or an excruciating, shooting, throbbing, mind-blowing pain,
or the WORST headache they ever had.

it is true for some,
but not for everyone.
I did not have any of that.
a blood vessel opened, but no pain,
a whoosh from a leaky blood vessel,
the burst was a feather, floating to earth,
landing in a strange place.
it was a powerful and a quiet crash

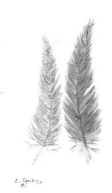

(Permission to use granted by artist, Ed Good)

CHAPTER 5

I Love Crepes. *J'adore les crêpes.*

February 2, 2015
Morning One, Week Two – End of Hospital Stay
Inpatient Rehabilitation (IP Rehab)

Food

AT every meal, I was given a menu to fill out for the next meal's menu. I could not understand what I was reading. I had to use my left hand to check what foods I wanted. At each meal, I never remembered what I ordered. I thought I was ordering French toast, but whatever it was, it was pureed. I was able to chew and swallow but, like many stroke victims, it took a few days for my swallow reflex to strengthen. To qualify for solid foods, my swallow reflex to be fully intact. When my menu was upgraded to chopped foods, someone had to cut up my food. It would be 10 months before I used a knife with my right hand.

> **Health Tip:** If your doctor tells you to cut out salt, sweets, high cholesterol foods for health reasons, do it. If you end up in the hospital, your meals will be monitored by a dietician who follows doctor's instructions. The dietician will not give you something the doctor says you cannot have.

I have always been a very picky eater. I make no secret of the foods that I dislike.

- Brussels sprouts
- cooked cabbage
- lima beans
- cherries
- the list goes on and on

Foods that I like, but was not on the list of foods that I could have:

- eggs
- salads
- saltine crackers
- decaf coffee
- peaches
- applesauce
- cream
- milk

Nothing was appealing. The food did not taste good. There were odd sensations: metallic, very salty, strange tastes, lingering unpleasantly in my mouth. I could not come up with the words to describe it. The nurses and my family encouraged me to eat even if the food did not taste good. I bellyached and complained. My family was sorry I disliked the food, but they believed complaining about the food meant that I was feeling better.

Most people think hospital food is not tasty. I worked at this hospital; the food was good, very good. A snack room was open to families. My husband always found something, such as ice cream. He said everything tasted fine. My appetite was gone. I was never hungry. I did not even want my favorite cheesy potatoes. The old tastes did not return for six months; the metallic taste was gone. The first taste back was sour, then bitter, then salty. Sweets and chocolate came back at 18 months.

Two years post-stroke, we were in Paris. I had a crepe on the first day and delicious croissants every day. My appetite was back and I was hungry.

Tip: Caution! Do not make people eat foods they do not like. My brother, Jeff, did not like peas; I didn't either. Peas were soft and mushy. I gagged and spit them out. My little brother had to sit at the table all evening, until bedtime, until the peas were colder, softer, and mushier. When he got up in the morning, those colder, softer and mushier peas were waiting for him. As an adult, he discovered he was allergic to peas.

February 2 - 9, 2015
First week and Second Week
Inpatient Rehabilitation (IP Rehab)
Activities of Daily Living (ADL)

Spoons and ADL

A spoon is a spoon unless it is an adapted, therapeutic tool used to help me regain skills so I could feed myself. If I could not feed myself, what else can I not do? The answer is a number of things. I was able to use a spoon or fork with my left hand. My right arm and hand were weak. My right hand could not operate a spoon. An adaptive spoon was weighted and strapped around my right hand. The diminished sensation in my right hand made me unaware that there was a spoon in my hand. So why would I put an adaptive spoon in my right hand? That is easy. It is the first step to regaining strength, function, and independence.

Steps to use my right hand:

- Use left hand to feed self.

- Sit on my left hand.

- Strap a weighted spoon onto right hand.

- Wrap fingers around the strap on right hand.

- Take the spoon to the plate, pick up food, and take food to my mouth using right hand.

- Pay attention to what I was doing.

When I turned my head to the left, my right hand, and my brain would forget that I was holding a spoon. The spoon and food would drop to the table or ground. It was amazing; I learned about that when I was in occupational therapy classes. What do you think about that? The helper in the dining room told me that she would get me more food. "It's okay," she said, cheerfully every time. I am grateful to the people who picked up the food I dropped. They did not want me to be embarrassed. I was not embarrassed, but it was nice that they cared about my feelings. I do not want to forget the people who prepared the food. It was not their fault that I hated the food. I am indebted to the therapists who taught me every task in achievable steps.

I love crepes, but there were no crepes in the hospital cafeteria. J'adore les crêpes, mais il n'y a pas de crêpes à la cafétéria de l'hôpital. (Please note: I was not able to speak French fluently after the stroke or before. Thank you, Google Translator.)

February 2 to February 9, 2015
Week Two, Three, Four
Inpatient Rehabilitation (IP Rehab)
Occupational Therapy (OT), Physical Therapy (PT, Speech Therapy (ST),
Social Work (SW) and Rest (Rest)

What the heck are PT, OT, ST, SW, and all the rest of the alphabet professions?

TWO signs should be posted in every OT, PT, and ST Clinic. When you enter: "Caution: All your powers will not magically reappear after one session of therapy." When you exit: "To do any of the activities, everything takes as long as it takes." On day two of therapies, I discovered that I had a quiet earthquake in my brain. The stroke was an equal opportunity attacker; it affected fine and gross motor skills, the senses, and cognition. But the hopeful part of this condition is that I was surrounded by smart people who were ready to help me. Every person helped me with one or two little things and all I had to do was to accept their assistance.

I have been a patient in Physical Therapy in this hospital before, once for a sore back and once after I broke my right leg, the tibia and fibula. I had surgery to hold the bones together with screws and clamps, six weeks in a cast, followed by six weeks of physical therapy. A broken leg is noticeable. A stroke is invisible. A broken leg is humbling and inconvenient, but time and therapy enabled me to get back on the road. One teeny, broken capillary and my life was turned upside down.

The total effect of aphasia and right-sided weakness would become obvious during the first days of therapy. I answered questions with yes and no, but often I was not sure if the answer was yes or no. I had difficulty following directions and I was extremely tired. In therapy, I had to re-learn everything, including things I could do in kindergarten. I learned once and I could learn it again, but I learned faster when I was 4 or 5 than I did at sixty three and sixty nine.

If someone told me I was not competent or I was not doing things well, that did not make me feel poorly. I understood that I was in a therapy room on a rehabilitation unit because I was not able to do anything well. It was not a failure. Therapy is the place that I started. As soon as I accomplished one thing, I moved on to something else that I could not do … yet. Cross Country runners strive for their "Personal Best." Me, too.

February 2 to February 20, 2015
Inpatient Rehabilitation (IP Rehab)
Occupational Therapy (OT), Physical Therapy (PT), Speech Therapy (ST)

Therapists & Therapy

I like Therapy—OT, PT, ST, all of it. I am half patient and half Occupational Therapist. I never expected a therapist to be perfect; I expected them to share their knowledge. PT and OT sessions last an hour each. Speech Therapy is split into two half-hour sessions. PT and OT are more physical. I never would have been able to tolerate an hour of Speech. Speech Therapy was particularly unsettling. I was given worksheets that I received in kindergarten and first grade. I could not complete them.

Therapy is not child's play, little kids' stuff. My age did not determine what I needed. My specific deficits guided what needed to be done as my brain and body were healing so I could regain skills. I attended therapy every day, but after the first day, I was not my old chipper, perky self. I never had a temper tantrum saying, "I am never coming back." I never stomped out of a session because I could not walk without assistance. I was living in the moment. I was not thinking if I did better than the day before or if I would do better tomorrow. I did not even think how I would do the next hour. I just showed up.

Good Words and Sounds, aka Affirmations

I required ongoing reminders and verbal cues from the therapist while I was working. I used little helpful sayings to help me when I was frustrated, affirmations like The Little Engine's "I think I can. I think I can." These little pep talks have always been a part of my routine.

When I learned to use a spoon with my right hand, it was a challenge. I used Affirmations and Good Words to keep me focused. I used these phrases over and over again in rehabilitation, in-patient and out-patient. Affirmations and Good Words are more powerful if they make me giggle:

- Good Words #1: "I learned everything when I was little. I can learn everything again."

- Good Words #2: "Enough for now. Rest."

- Good Words #3: "I am doing the best that I can."

- Good Words #4: "I CANNOT do it … yet."

- Good Words #5: "I do not wish for changes. I make changes."

- Super Good Words #6: "Stop. I did it. On to the next task."

- Good Words #7: At the end of an activity, "Thank you" to the therapist, yourself, and anyone standing by your side.

- Good Words #8: "I move through life vertically with ease and grace."

- Good Words #9: "Keep walking. Keep doing everything."

1957

Affirmations and Hereafters

MISS Smart was my first, second, and third teacher. Miss Smart had a little library in our classroom. She told me that when I finished my work and if I did not talk to my neighbors during class, I could go into the library and read all the books I wanted. There was no library in the fourth- and fifth-grade classroom, which led to talking to my neighbors and being regularly assigned to write "Hereafters."

Instructions: "On a piece of paper, please write, 'Hereafter, I will not talk to my neighbors during class' twenty five times. Please write your name in the top right-hand corner."

Twenty five times would become fifty times, then one hundred and possibly five hundred times. Sometimes I was invited to write on the chalkboard during class.

It really did not matter who my neighbor was, I could find something interesting to talk with a classmates about during class. I found writing "Hereafters" creative and therapeutic. I wrote the first 25 with my right hand and the next 25 with my left. I wrote the next 25 starting at the bottom of the page. The next 25 would be in red. "Hereafters" taught me about time management. No matter how many "Hereafters" I was assigned, I could always finish in time for recess.

I eventually discovered why I should not talk to my neighbors during class. It was distracting and disrespectful. I learned this very important lesson just as I was going into sixth grade. Coincidentally, the sixth-, seventh-, and eighth-grade room had an attached library. No more "Hereafters."

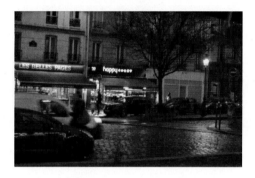

(Happy in Paris / Heureux à Paris)

Thoughts

Hereafter, I will not talk to my neighbors during therapy sessions

When I was in grade school, I often wrote,
"Hereafter, I will not talk to my neighbors during class."

When I was in therapy, I never wrote,
"Hereafter, I will not talk to my neighbors during therapy sessions"
because I was not aware of anyone else in the therapy clinic
and the others didn't notice me.

Instead, I wrote,
"Hereafter, I will monitor my blood pressure once a day,
every day,"

And then I wrote,
"Hereafter, I will use my right hand to write,"
five times a day or as tolerated.

And then I wrote,
"Hereafter, I will take the train to Chicago by myself,"
as many times until I take the train all by myself.

And then I wrote,
"Hereafter, I will fly to Sioux Falls, South Dakota
and change planes in Chicago all by myself,"
until I fly back and forth to Sioux Falls by myself, with special assistance.

And then I wrote,
"Hereafter, I will go to Paris" or "Par la suite, j'irai à Paris,"
a thousand times until I go to Paris,
a thousand times until I return to Paris.

Hereafter, I will not talk to my neighbors during therapy.
Hereafter, I will not talk to my neighbors during therapy.
Hereafter, I will use my right hand to write.

Hereafter, I will use my right hand to write.
Hereafter, I will go to Paris.
Hereafter, I will go to Paris again.
Hereafter, I will go to Paris and again.
Hereafter, I will go to Paris and again.
Hereafter, I will go to Paris and again.
Hereafter, I will go to Paris and again.
Hereafter, I will go to Paris and again.
Hereafter, I will go to Paris and again.
Hereafter, I will go to Paris and again.

CHAPTER 6

Camp

February 2 to February 6, 2015
February 9 to February 13, 2015
February 15 to February 20, 2015
In-Patient Rehabilitation (Rehab)
Physical Therapy and Physical Therapist (PT)

Camp Rehab: PT

I arrived at the therapy clinic on the first day of rehabilitation. The tasks I performed during my first therapy session were completed with assistance and very slowly.

- stand

- walk to therapy table

- turn around

- sit down

- stand up

- repeat as tolerated

The Physical Therapist used verbal cues, repeated, as needed. She supported me physically, even when I was sitting. I could not lean on my right hand /arm to hold me up; I was weak and wobbly. The next task:

- stand

- walk to therapy table

- turn around

- sit down on therapy table

- lay down

- sit up
- lay down
- roll to side
- roll on to tummy
- roll back to side
- onto back
- sit up
- stand

I don't think I did all of the steps more than two times until the second week. When I was on my back or rolling to my side, I rested at each step. Being able to get up on all fours and holding that position was rigorous:

- lay on back
- roll to side
- roll to laying on tummy
- get up on all hands and knees
- slowly lower myself on tummy
- roll to side
- lay on back

I repeated these movements until I "mastered them" and / or till I could do them a couple of times and then move on to something new. Every day, I could do a wee bit more with less assistance, but I had some assistance the entire time I was at the hospital. Going up and down stairs was such a challenge because I could not remember what foot to start with. I was the kid who was always told, "Slow down, patience." I finally listened. I have patiently slowed down.

The PT stood by my side and told me what to do. She helped me as needed and encouraged me. She told me that I have improved and how I improved. I continued with the exercises as long as I could. I was comfortable telling all of the therapists—PT, OT, ST—when I needed to rest or stop. I definitely did not use affirmations the first week, maybe not even the second or third week. My affirmations remained simple: "Okay." It would take time until my movements flowed smoothly. By the end of three weeks, I could walk alone with a walker, with a therapist close enough to prevent me from falling.

Physical Therapists know everything.

I took tap dancing lessons when I was 3, 4, and 5 years old. I loved my tap shoes and the noise. I was not very skilled; I could only use my right foot to do the soft shoe move, never my left foot. Wearing tap shoes to walk might be helpful because I will hear when I drag my right foot.

February 2 to February 6, 2015
February 9 to February 13, 2015
February 15 to February 20, 2015
In Patient Rehabilitation (IP Rehab)
Occupational Therapy and Occupational Therapist (OT)

Camp Rehab: OT

IN order for my mind and body to return to my control, I had to start over, doing everything a lot like a baby. My muscles were weak and I was unsteady standing, moving, and sitting. I didn't have any idea of how to move. My left hand compensated for my right hand automatically. My ability to think and process instructions was muddled. Verbal instructions were confusing; I could only process one instruction at a time. The therapist would have to demonstrate what she wanted me to do, over and over. When I returned to therapy the next day, I had to have the instructions repeated. I was fortunate that I didn't become discouraged. I had been a very organized person, but everything now felt disorganized. If my eyes were closed and I was lying down, I could not determine if my right arm was at a 90-degree angle or laying flat on the bed.

Occupational Therapists use activities and techniques that address right-side body awareness, as well as fine motor skills, balance, movement, coordination, strengthening muscles, and increasing agility. Using simple movements, reaching across the middle of the body, send cues to the brain to reconnect the left and right sides of my brain. To improve fine motor skills, involving the small muscles in fingers, thumb and hands, as well as eye – hand coordination with right hand:

- Pick up a clothes pin from a basket. Open it and then hang it on a basket placed on my left side.
- Pick up pennies in the sand, set them down on my left side. It seems simple, but it took several attempts.
- Repeat.

- To improve gross motor skills, the large muscles, body awareness, and coordination of left and right side of body, strengthen core muscles, and prevent shoulder droop and injuries, good body mechanics, range of motion was necessary. Movements and exercises are invaluable. Here are just a few that I could do early on:

- cross arms and legs and hand

- patty cake

- hug yourself

- say a prayer

- look left to right, up and down

- pass a ball from left side to right

Who am I and where am I? I know what city is? I know what building I am in. I know that I am a patent in a hospital that I used to work in. The employees have name tags. If I ever go back to school to become a doctor, my thesis will be "Proprioception". Discovering where in the world am I?"

Occupational Therapists Know Everything.

February 2 to February 6, 2015
February 9 to February 13, 2015
February 15 to February 20, 2015
In Patient Rehabilitation (I-P Rehab)
Speech Therapy and Speech Therapist (ST)

Camp Rehab: ST

MOST of my conversations were simple and initiated by others. "How are you feeling?" "How was your dinner?" My sentences were not complex or complete, often making it difficult for the listener to understand what I was trying to say. My listeners were willing to figure it out without making me use the right words. I would have the words eventually. I needed to be listened to. I could speak and hear, but communication with others took a back seat to all the work I had to do in the Speech Therapy clinic.

The Speech Therapist (ST) used activities to address the different areas of difficulty. The ST showed me a card with pictures of two items, turned it over, then asked, "Can you tell me which two items were on this card?" Although hesitating, I still answered correctly. I did it!

The ST showed me a card with three items, and turned it over, "Can you tell me the three items that were on this card?" Sometimes I could do it and sometimes I could not. So I'd try again.

The ST repeated the instructions, "This time, four items." Think. Think. Think. Breathe. Looking at the back of the card, closing my eyes. If I had to recall four items I could not remember even one item. I knew that someday I would be able to recall all four of them. I did whatever I needed to do in speech therapy even if I never improved.

Being able to name all four items on the cards, I had to giggle. The Speech Therapist would have been impressed to know how many things I could remember when I was 7. One goal I had in Speech Therapy was to be able to finish a sentence, at least sometimes. I had to take it easy on myself. Some of the most memorable conversations I have ever had, occurred when a group of friends got together. Laughter and interrupted conversations.

Speech Therapists know everything.

Thoughts

a stroke is a brain injury,
a dark light,
resulting in brain damage.

just Words
"disabling",
just Words
"bruised and wounded",
just Words
"weak and slow and clumsy",
just Words
"fear",
just Words
are not just Words.

I prefer helpful Words.
I prefer hopeful Words.
"not forever",
"slowly improving", "healing",
"moving", "mobile".

a handicapped parking tag
and special assistance means
I have places to go,
every day places,
the places I dream of.
I will move through the day with ease and grace.
These are the Words that I like.

just Words
"all by myself".

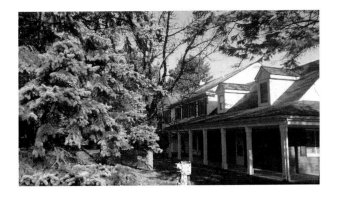

CHAPTER 7

GOING HOME

Happy Trails

THE first thing I saw when I opened my eyes two days after I arrived at the hospital was my family. Every day, my family was there. Even with a fine medical team, the most positive thing for my recovery was family. They supported and encouraged me to stay on task. That was good.

My medical team said I would be doing much better in six months. They stressed I would continue to improve after that. Loving friends and family said, "In six months, you'll be good as new." They told me this over and over with love and hope. They loved the old me. Those are the words they should say, but I did not want to be my old self. My old self had a few cracks. My body has had many bumps and broken places over the years because I was always in a hurry and I didn't pay attention. This stroke, this one teeny, broken blood vessel was a warning. This was the opportunity to fix what needed to be tweaked and fixed; both my physical self and mind can and will make healthier choices. When I was young, playing outside, I fell down, fell of my bike, climbed trees, even if the branches were shaky, and I just kept playing. I would put band aids on scrapes and went back out and played. Everyone, at every age, needs to take care of their one and only body. After the stroke, I discovered for myself how salt increased my blood pressure. I could see the numbers on a blood pressure cuff and compare how I felt, headache and out of sorts. It's silly. I have always known the connection of salt and high blood pressure. I thought I controlled the amount of salt I used, but sadly, I didn't do a very good job. Salt is in so many foods. I have gone back to reading labels and drink more water.

My husband had a pragmatic view of what I could and could not do. Every day he told me specifically how I was getting better. That was magic. It was the frosting on the cake, with candles, waiting for me to blow them out. Of course, you are not allowed to have burning candles in the hospital and I would not have been able to blow them out anyway.

Still, it was magic. My husband only said what he could observe. He did not know about the future. He did not know how much I would be able to do and how long it would take. There was so much that I had to do, would fail to do and try again. My family stood by my side and helped me until I could do things all by myself.

I had a car accident in 1971. I flipped my beloved 1969 Mustang, end over end, rolling it until we it landed on the roof. I was not hurt; I crawled out through the window, and ran to a nearby house to call the police. Someone else called the police, too. Poor little car. At that moment, I thought maybe a repair truck could just flip it over and I could drive home. Sad me. It took between 6 and 8 weeks to fix. It was not quite as good as new, but it got me to where I had to go.

People occasionally tell me they would never know I had a stroke. That is their kindness talking. Early on you could tell that I had not been well, but the outside bounces back faster than the inside. The better they know me, the more they know I am not quite as good as I used to be, but I can get to where I have to go.

Thank you, Dale Evans, for writing one of my favorite songs, "Happy Trails to you". Thank you for making it cool to be a cowgirl.

February 21, 2015

Camp Home

I went home. I had to sleep downstairs for two weeks before I slept in my own bed. Our kitties were glad I was home. Flora, our black-with-white-markings cat, meowed at me. Loretta, our white-with-black-markings cat, slept on my right arm all night for weeks. I had to have somebody with me the first two weeks after I returned home. Even after the two weeks, I was not alone for quite a long time. People stopped by, kept me company, or took me to therapy. And they kept me from being afraid.

My nieces, Elizabeth and Hannah, spent a few days with me. We watched HGTV and discussed which house was our favorite, our favorite show, and who I wanted to renovate and decorate my house; it was Joanna and Chip Gaines, of course. Hannah and Elizabeth made me lunch, exactly what I wanted and exactly the way I wanted it. It was delicious and it was the first meal I enjoyed since

January 26. This delicious meal and watching HGTV made this one of my happiest days. I was thankful for what they did, but the feeling I was having was love for these two girls. I don't know if Elizabeth and Hannah know that. This is what Elizabeth and Hannah did for me that day:

- made lunch and dinner
- cut up my own food
- fed the cats
- washed my hair
- gather my clothes for the day
- went grocery shopping
- did the laundry
- answered the phone

Hitchhiking

THANKS to my friends, Ruth Martin and Diane Bogenrieder, for picking me up and driving me to therapy sessions and other places I needed to go. Thanks, because they were good company, and it gave my husband the chance to go back to work, and I didn't have to hitchhike.

A Week Post Hospital Discharge (PHD)

Doctors, Nurses, Navigators

A few days after I was discharged from the hospital, I had an appointment with my primary care physician to plan for follow-up care. I was assigned nurse managers through my primary care physician and insurance companies. They provided referrals to other services, including OT, PT, ST and Social Worker.

I needed to be seen by a neurologist. My primary care physician gave me options. When I decided which neurologist I wanted to see, my physician made the appointment. I went to the neurologist a few weeks later. She performed an assessment, asked me and my husband a lot of questions. She was very thorough, explaining where I was at the beginning, how far I had come, my expectations, and my husband's expectations. She listened and explained until we understood and our questions were answered. The same was true for my primary care physician and the nurses. They kept me from getting lost.

I wanted to go to a Social Worker. The nurse made a list of candidates. It included specialties, location, and time preferences. She presented choices and when I decided, she made the appointment for me. She followed up to make sure I was satisfied with the therapist I chose.

One to Three Months Post Hospital Discharge (PHD)

Thank Goodness for Gadgets

KEEPING in touch with the outside world was difficult. My smart phone and computer connected me to anyone I wanted to talk to, but I could not remember how to use them. For the first two or three months at home, I was too tired to talk on the phone, even for a few minutes. Writing was, and still is, a challenge. When I started to use my computer, I typed with my left hand and moved the mouse with my left hand. Gadgets and tools kept me in contact with the outside world. For the time being, most people I knew lived in the outside world.

Communication had been important to me, ever since I was little. I am curious and nosy. Before I got a princess phone in my room, I had to use the phone in the middle of the family room. Not ideal, but I could pull the six-foot phone cord from the family room, down the hall and into a closet. The day I got a princess phone in my room was a national holiday! If I could go back in time and change one thing, it would be to never call a phone "Princess." If I had known about Ruth Bader Ginsburg then, I would have insisted on a RBG Supreme Court phone.

Google was useful. I could type in a few words and it knew what I wanted. It would be nice if people could be as helpful. Keywords, not a complete sentence, and you can find whatever you need on Google. And whoever created the Microsoft Office, "Find" and "Cut and Paste" features was a genius. Everyone looks for the newest gadget and improved technology. Me, too. AutoCorrect makes me cranky, but I am confident that there will be improvements. Some think that aphasia is a disability. No, it's an early version that will improve with time, maybe quicker than AutoCorrect is updated. I did a little research as to what caused more frustration: AutoCorrect or aphasia. My research showed that AutoCorrect caused considerably more frustration. It was overwhelmingly AutoCorrect. Who was in the research group? Me.

It would not have been possible to write this story, whether by hand or using a computer, without therapy and gadgets. Therapy helped me weave my motor and cognitive skills back together again; the gadgets helped me make things pretty. One of my first jobs was as an operator on a PBX Switchboard. I learned how to answer calls and when to disconnect, a useful life lesson.

Six Weeks Post Stroke (PS) –Year Five, Ongoing
Outpatient Rehabilitation (OP Rehab)
Occupational Therapy (OT)

OT

AN Occupational Therapist (OT) evaluated my skills before I started driving again. I dreamed about driving when I was 7 or 8. By the time I received my license at 16, I was ready. This time I was unsure what to expect. It was more than seven months until I drove. Think of all the steps that had to be coordinated in order to drive. It was daunting. I followed all the rules of the road. Primarily, I drove down Ann Arbor Trail to downtown Plymouth—roughly two miles and very light traffic. No cruising down Main Street. It was a long time till I drove with a friend in the car, no texting, no talking on the phone. I know how teenagers feel, but it was a good rule for me.

An OT suggested that I needed to protect my right side from injury and my left side from overuse. She advised me to return to therapy every year for a little tune-up. It was valuable advice and it is still true. Four years looking down at the ground while walking so I would not fall left my posture in a sorry state. Now the goal is to strengthen my core so I stand tall with good posture. Continuing in OT and PT, I feel I am making progress. It was not that long ago that I could not walk by myself. Ta Da!

Eight Weeks Post Stroke (PS)
Outpatient Rehabilitation (OP Rehab)
Speech Therapy (ST)

OP Rehab Speech Therapy (ST): Aphasia, Squirrels, Birds, Groundhogs, Deer, and Bunnies

I could not easily retrieve words or images; that is how aphasia manifested in me. I could recall plots of books, but when I attempted to retell the story, I struggled to find the words to do so. The Speech Therapist gave me an activity to name all the animals I could think of in one minute. To make this more relevant, she suggested I start with the animals in my yard. I closed my eyes, breathed deeply and visualized my yard. I counted to 10. Ready? Go.

- "Squirrels"
- "Birds"
- *Think think think:* "Groundhogs"
- *I can't see my animals.*
- *Someone stole all my animals.*

That was it. Squirrels, birds, and a couple of groundhogs and I could not even name the type of bird. I did not see any more animals, no deer, no bunnies, and no blue jays. My words were not there and now the pictures were gone, too. Pine trees, burning bushes, and lilacs disappeared. My reaction was wow; aphasia is a big deal. The enormity of how the stroke impacted me was clear. By this time, however, I had made progress in different ways that bolstered my confidence. I was adamant that I continue to regain skills and improve my ability to find words and name things. I did not want to lose the critters and plants in my yard ever again. I still fumble for words; I just have to close my eyes and reach in and grab them.

At four and a half years post stroke, I intended to type the word "Hummingbird." Instead, I typed "Hemingbird." Maybe I was thinking of Hummingbirds and dreaming of Hemingway and Paris.

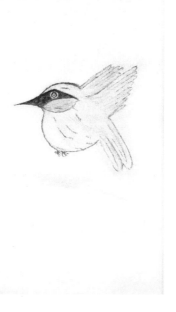

(Permission to use granted by artist, Ed Good)

It is not necessary to stop the person who has aphasia and correct them. Let them say what they want to say. Do not stop them mid-sentence and point out the errors in their speech. They did not say anything wrong; their brain just made a different choice. Did you get the gist of what they were trying to say? Listen to the way they talk, the rhythm. Move through their world for a few minutes. You do not have to guess; you can always ask.

Babies cannot talk, but often you can figure out what they want. Listen to a baby, a young child. It is not what they say that is so important; it is that the adults in their life teach them how to listen to others. Do you know what your dog or cat is saying to you? Animals are patient with their humans. Talk and listen with your heart, ears, eyes, face, and touch. Listening with gentleness is powerful and will help the one with aphasia; it may benefit the listener, too.

Three Weeks Post Hospital Discharge (PHD)

UTI

A simple little UTI (Urinary Tract infection), aka Hell, and I was back in the hospital. I was very sick. My speech was more garbled than it was the first few days after the stroke. It was frightening, but the doctor said that once the infection cleared up, my speech may return. Two nights in the hospital, a course of antibiotics and my speech returned as it was two days before. I found a very helpful urologist to help me get off the UTI roller coaster. Thank goodness. I did not ask anyone why the doctor said my speech "may return."

I could say more, but that is all for now.

Three Weeks - Six Months Post Stroke (PS)

Anything Else?

WHEN I was in the hospital, everyone was focused on getting me up and moving around. I did not get a good case of the weepies and anxiety until I went home, to the real world. I was on an emotional roller coaster for about four months. I dealt with emotional issues, tears, fear, sadness, and depression. I believe that continued therapy and support from family and friends guided me, like a collie, as I worked through the panic attacks quickly and with less severity. I had never had them before, but I understood what was happening. A Social Worker taught me techniques to fight panic attacks and addressed the impact of all that had occurred to me for the past few months. It was very impactful to work with therapists, OT, PT, ST, and Social Workers who addressed my body issues and emotional health.

A friend, Mike Maloney, told me, "Take things a day at a time." My response was, "How about five minutes at a time?"

Don't underestimate the power of another person reaching out to you. My friend, Jennifer Arapoff, sent me a text: "When are you up for an Arapoff Girls visit?" The way I felt at the time, I probably would have said "no," but the Arapoff girls were the perfect medicine for what ailed me. After their visit, I felt relieved. Thank you, Julia, Alexa, Anna, Jennifer Arapoff, and Kathy Powers for cheering me up. That was the end of panic attacks and the gloominess…almost.

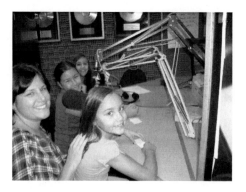

(The Arapoff's being interviewed at WSDP,
Permission to use granted by Jennifer Arapoff)

More Children

THE summer of 2015, I needed a ride to everywhere. It never bothered me, but on Wednesdays I was happy in Kellogg Park at "Music in the Park". I got to hang with Ayla and her mom, Tricia Kennedy, Leah and Molly and their super nanny, Rachel Koelzer. Jamie Jones and her clan always had room on their blankets for me to share: Mason, Alexa, Skylar, Gavin, Stella, and the adults, Sue and Dave Jones. Megan and Brendon Weil, Kevin and Kendra Jones. I still moved slow and deliberate, but the lovely children around me danced to the music. It was a happiness explosion that was helping my brain wake up to the world around me. Children animate my world and fill my heart and mind with joy.

Three Months Post Stroke (PS), Ongoing

There was one more surprise! Chronic Post Stroke Pain (CPSP)

THREE months post-stroke, out of nowhere, I had tingling on the right side of my body. Over the course of a week to 10 days, the tingling became more pronounced and constant. I was alarmed. What began as tingling on my right side increased from irritating to uncomfortable, escalating to a burn, and then pain. My blood pressure was okay and I had no other symptoms of a stroke.

I called my primary care physician. She listened carefully to the symptoms I was experiencing. She consulted with the neurologist. The neurologist contacted me. I described my symptoms; she made an appointment for me to see her as soon as possible. Going back to the neurologist was scary, but my fear faded when the neurologist identified what was causing the pain and the available treatments. What had been so scary was that no one had mentioned this possibility.

The neurologist explained that she thought this pain / irritation was Chronic Post Stroke Pain (CPSP), Central Post Stroke Pain or Constant Neuropathic Pain. Right Side CPSP appeared, out of nowhere. No, it did not really appear out of nowhere. It originated in the thalamus, basal ganglia the spot injured by the CVA. The neurologist explained that due to the area of the brain where I had a hemorrhagic stroke, it is more common to have Chronic Post Stroke Pain, occurring four to six months post-stroke. CPSP does not affect all stroke patients.

I experienced CPSP on my right side; it was most notable in my hand and foot. The neurologist discussed medications that may be helpful. The one I chose has been effective. At a certain dose, the medication alleviated the pain almost completely, but it made me sleep for almost twelve hours. Lowering the dosage, the discomfort was mildly irritating. I tried to go off the medication completely, but that was painful and I was very cold. The pain consumed me so I could not focus on anything else. Appling lotions to my arm and leg did not help because all the sensations / messages were coming from the brain. Fortunately, the discomfort has not interfered with sleep.

It was reassuring that even though my communication skills were affected, I understood what was being explained to me. Note: no more surprises, please.

When I walked, it felt like I had a new, never used, full-sized sanitary napkin on the bottom of my right foot. It felt like I was walking in a rocking boat. This has improved over the years. Now it feels like a new, never used, panty liner under my toes and heel and a thick pad in the middle of my right foot. My right hand feels like I plunged it into a cake with coconut frosting and then put it into the freezer for awhile. And upon removing it from the freezer, I separated my sticky, still-frozen, fingers. Today, my fingers are thawing.

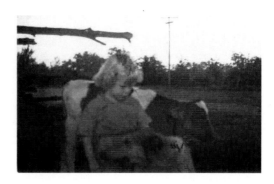

Juggling

WHEN my children were babies, I carried them, shifting from side to side. The baby and I had our own rhythm. When I had a second baby, the baby's rhythm did not quite match Baby #1's rhythm. Going grocery shopping with Baby #1 and Baby #2 was physically and mentally challenging—running after one baby, calmly rocking the other baby, and getting everything on my shopping list all at the same time. My boat was rocking. Post-stroke, my left side is the quiet, calm and mellow me. My right side is more active, noisier and demands all my attention. Another way to describe the two sides is the left side naps and the right side is on LSD Acid-Lite.

My right side could not predict the weather, storms or rain. My right side did not know when the moon was full or waning. But when it was cold, my right side grabbed a megaphone and shouted, "I am very cold." It was not like holding an icicle; it was an overall achiness. Hot weather did not affect me. I had to be careful when I picked up a cup or plate that was hot or cold with my right hand. It took me a few seconds to react. When I swam, I did not tolerate cold water and I could not think of anything else. When the water was warm, it was as comfortable and relaxing as if I were sleeping.

In addition to the temperature being affected by CPSP, my right hand has sensory distortion. If I hold a soft sweater, it may looks like it is soft; but it feels like fine sandpaper. It may be an inconvenience, but it also a loss. When I touch someone's face, a child's hair or a soft kitty with my right hand, I could cry. But I can switch to my left hand quickly and the crying stops.

Chronic Post Stroke Pain (CPSP)

I am sure you have seen the Pain Scale: Happy Face to Angry Face. This scale does not apply to me. I experience tingling, not pain, irritation, not pain. Smiles or sad faces do not describe what I am feeling. Nerve pain is experienced by many people, not just those with CPSP. It only applies to my right side, especially my right hand.

This is my Irritation Scale.

1. No sensory discomfort, sleeping

2. Waking

3. Dull tingling

4. Scratchy

5. Sandpaper

6. Chilly

7. Not able to ignore when the sensations in my fingers and hands when writing and typing with my right hand. The longer I type or write, my fingers get "stuck", really "stuck". My thumb and index finger aren't impaired, but my other three don't bend easily. I have to use my left hand to assist picking up a spoon, pen, and chopsticks. Without my middle finger, I am not very proficient.

8. Am I the only person who can load the dirty dishes into the dishwasher? Am I the only person who can start the dishwasher? Am I the only person who can put the clean dishes away? (This should not be on this list, but it is irritating.)

9. Thawing out hours after being frozen

10. Thawing out immediately after being frozen

11. Frostbite and freezing, cannot find relief

Three Years Post Stroke (PS), Ongoing
Social Work / Social Worker (SW)

The Pause

I am familiar with social workers, therapists, counselors, and their role in health care. I was impressed with my social worker, an extremely kind woman, compassionate, a listener, and a keen observer. We all may need to put our pieces back together again from time to time, even though we are chipped and many of the pieces do not fit together.

This social worker listened as I sorted through and came to understand the changes that I was going through, assess how I coped with them, and find the path where I wanted the next steps to take me. I have fallen down many times, popped back up, and told everyone, "I am fine", and continued on my way. Sometimes, I did not pop back up, but I still told everyone, "I am fine". I thought this strategy worked. It did, and then, it did not anymore. I was lost, travelling in a big circle, and I did not even notice. It would have been a better idea to stay on the ground and make sure I was okay first. First responders know that people tell them they are okay, but they are not. After a physical injury or distress, people are in a fog, in shock.

When I awoke after the stroke, I just wanted to do whatever I had to do to get back to my life quickly. This time was different. I could say "I am fine" all day long, but I was not going anywhere. I was caught. My counselor gave me uninterrupted time, which I learned to use wisely. She made the space safe and I committed to listening when she spoke. I trusted her and I trusted myself.

She made sure she understood what she heard, what I said, and what I meant. She had the knack for asking the right questions and when I started to answer, I could not come up with any words. I had to stop and think about what she asked and then think some more. At that moment, I knew what we were talking about was important and serious. This time, there was no "I am fine" and escaping. This counselor introduced me to taking a "pause." And she was right there while I learned how.

Too often I wanted to flee. I did not want to sit down and be still, even when I did not accomplish anything. I was hesitant to face something I thought better forgotten…because…I…did…not…want…to…remember. I wanted to get back to my life. I paced back and forth until I was right in the middle of a trauma that may have taken place one year ago or fifty years ago. I found myself in that place I never wanted to be. But with the support of the social worker, I now had an exit strategy. I took a moment to think, rested my weary brain, and body. I had the ability to walk all the way up and through the trauma. I used words to examine the trauma. I was given the opportunity for a course correction, maybe change the world or change myself, and it did not take forever.

When it was time to wrap up with the social worker, she said to call her any time. I knew she did not mean to call and we would go to lunch because we were now friends. I will be grateful for meeting and working with this woman forever. I have met many gifted people who have the skills to support a person confront difficult situations. They are those rare individuals who want nothing more than for you to be well, not just "fine".

Medical caregivers are empathetic; they have the gift of knowing how to approach frightened people. Imagine, a 10-year-old girl in a hospital emergency room with a broken arm, waiting for the results of an x-ray. She tells everyone, "I am fine. I am fine" over and over. That broken arm hurts, but she would not change her story. She did not tell anyone her arm hurts. Several people talked to her. It is not that they did not care, but they were not the "right person" for that little girl.

When the "right person" comes into the room and sits down, she does not ask the little girl if her arm hurts or what happened to her arm. She introduced herself. She asked the little girl what her name is, what school she goes to, her friends' names. The "right person" wanted to take care of the little girl's arm, but she knows she had to wait until the little girl is safe.

What could frighten a little girl more than a broken arm? The "right person" may never know that, but she took care of the little girl and her arm. The little girl will always remember the lady in the hospital as big and strong. When the little girl grows up, she may run into this woman. Surprisingly, the woman is not big, she is little. The grown up girl will not notice the woman is frail. She will never forget the woman who took care of her broken arm and gave her a doll.

At Home, Books and Reading and Numbers

HOME from the hospital, I had a lot of time and piles of books waiting to be read. It is mind-boggling to pick up a book and understand each word, but not the meaning of a paragraph. What I read on Page Two stood alone from the words on Page One and Page 188. I read every word on every page, but I could not remember the details from page to page. No story, only words. I had the same issues with audio books. Aphasia interfered with comprehension, but that did not stop me from loving books: gardening books, children's books, picture books, and the library.

I developed strategies to improve my reading skills. Before I started a book, I turned all devices off, turned the lights on, and sat up straight. I read page 1, stop and stop, page 2. Stop. Then:

- Drink water.

- Breathe.

- Read and read more.

- Write and write more.

- Rest often. My brain needed a lot of rest, more than I gave my brain in the past.

- Go for a walk. Exercise.

- Have patience.

Writing and typing are still cumbersome and uncomfortable. I know what I want to say, but writing so it is understood by the reader takes time. It does not matter whether I am sending a birthday card or writing this story. There may still be grammatical errors, typographical errors or misspelled words in the wrong place. It is helpful for me to:

- write shorter sentences and paragraphs.

- write fewer words on a page, more white space, and pictures.

- write lists, use bullet points.

- capitalize key words.

- write more poetry than prose.

- write a combination of poetry and medical charting.

- check and recheck what I have written.

- step away from the desk.

- read what I have written out loud.

- ask for help; both Hemingway and Fitzgerald had editors, the same man, Max Perkins.

Numbers require a different approach. I still do not have any good plans. I just have to check, check, check. When I make a deposit at the bank, I often ask the cashier to confirm my deposit verbally. When I make an appointment, I write it on a piece of paper and enter the date in my phone. It is helpful to have doctors and dentists who send email reminders.

> October 2015. I finished the first novel I read, post 1/27/15, Anna Quindlen's book, *Alternate Side*. I loved it. Ta Da!

Tips for a Possible Extended Hospital Stay

IF you are going to be in a hospital for more than a month, ask your husband to please call:

- Gail Maloney. She can grab a few clothes from my closet for me. A couple of nice outfits will make me feel human.

- Jenny Wendel, my hairdresser / therapist for thirty years. I am sure she will come to the hospital and give me a haircut. It will make me feel perky.

- Chinese restaurant for takeout, because it tastes good. Marcel often drove long distances to get the best Chinese food whenever I was not feeling well. I've always been proficient using chopsticks, but my fine motor skills are not as they once were.

- Bonus Tip: Purchase a sweater or coat for me from Maggie and Me because that always makes me feel better. If you don't know what I would like, ask Maggie, Shelly or Alexandra, they know what I like.

I did not think about any of this when I was in the hospital. Why am thinking about this now? I can look back on having a stroke, a hospital stay, and still giggle.

Special gratitude to the Staff at St. Mary Mercy Hospital and my primary physician, therapists, nurses, lab technician at University of Michigan staff to watch over me and help me get the care and services that I needed.

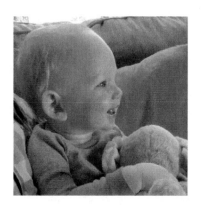

(Teddy. Permission to use granted by Andrew and Justine Madonna)

Thoughts

Hiding

my brain was filled with glorious, grandiose, splendid,
and sublime words and pictures.
my yard was home to creatures, flora, trees, bushes,
and squirrels that steal bird food.
no one understood how much I loved them all.

but
where was everyone?
where was everything?
I was going to write a letter to my brain, my yard,
and all who live here.
"where are you?
are you gone forever?
maybe you all will be home soon."

suddenly,
on the 5th of March,
on a sunny afternoon,
48 degrees,
3:37 p.m.,
the words came back,
not all.
the pictures in my mind came back,
not all.
the names in my mind came back.
not all at once,
almost all,
one at a time.

I am so happy to see you.
I have missed you so much,

even my mixed-up words missed you.
look who else came home:
trees, maple, apple, catalpas, pines blue, white,
flowers, lilacs, irises, mock orange, clay pots,
squirrels, bunnies, cardinals,
bluebirds, robins, hawks, deer,
groundhogs, opossum mothers and babies,
antlers shed by an 8-point buck,
and one lost kitty.

I took a leisurely walk later that day,
the 5th of March at 7:43 p.m.,
two deer were standing ten feet away,
maybe it was the deer that had shed this year's antlers.
perhaps they had been here all along,
with all the other animals and plants,
pictures and words.
Welcome Home, Dearest Friends.

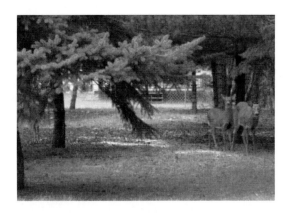

CHAPTER 8

Starting Over, Starting Together

Observing Growth & Development: Babies and Children, aka Teddy, and Me

HAVE you ever watched a baby doing something for the first time? Of course you have. Every day she does something new. Babies are these little balls of energy. We celebrate their milestones: first smile, first words. What skills does a baby have to master to take that first step? And once mastering that, she is on to the next skill. How do babies do all they do without a textbook or manual? Children need adequate nutrition. They need to trust the adults around them. Every child grows and develops at their own pace. We celebrate babies' and toddlers' accomplishments. Celebrating milestones should continue through elementary age, adolescence, adulthood, forever.

When a baby takes her first step, her audience watches, holds their breath, thinking, "You can do it." No matter how long that baby stands, 15 seconds or 5 seconds, the baby sees smiling faces. This response is repeated with every new skill. The first time I took a step after the stroke, I was shaky. While I was working to rebuild myself, I was not smiling. There was not always another face smiling back. A therapist gave me encouragement. Family and friends were supportive, but often they may have had a worried face, anxious, unsure. Remember even adults need a "Yippee", "Yahoo', "Ta Da", and a "You did it!"

Smile at a baby. Often they smile back without a lot of effort. Smile at a stroke survivor. You may try all your best tricks and jokes to get a smile. The stroke patient may be grinning inside, but the cheek muscles are not getting the message. The stroke patient may want to smile, but the small nerves may not be connected so that messages from the brain to the little muscles may not be getting through. Maybe the nerves to the muscles around the mouth and eyes were impacted by the stroke. I may intend to smile. I can part my lips, but there is no curve to it. How long will it take till they are working together again? I do not know.

I have always been a great crier over reality and fiction, books, movies, music, people, and Lassie. A few days ago, I was watching a movie, *A Dog Named Christmas* that I usually cry from the beginning to the end. I watched another movie that always makes me cry, sad and happy tears. At first I thought I had a tickle in my throat. That tickle became a full feeling in my chest and throat. I wondered if I was crying. There were no tears. The final test was to watch a Steve Hartman story, *On The Road, CBS Sunday Morning*, and not any particular story. Now I was sure it was tightening in my throat, quivering lips, warmth in the cheeks, and fullness in the lachrymal glands, and I was unable to speak. I had no tears, but everything else was there. I was satisfied, though, that this qualified as a good cry. I often feel like Mr. Spock or Data from Star Trek. I love them both, but I want my happiness to show.

When?

An obstetrician, a labor and delivery nurse, and all your friends can tell you the progression of labor. A pediatrician can assess whether a baby is meeting milestones. Children are surrounded by all sorts of experts, people who know about human growth and development. When I was pregnant with our sons, I had a lot of questions: "What is his due date?" "How long will my labor last?" The question I wanted to ask but could not ask was "Is my baby okay?"

After the stroke, the questions I had been: "Will I be able to walk?" "When will I be able to walk?" "Will I be able to speak and be understood?" "Will I be able to use my right hand to write a letter or use a fork and knife?" "Will I be able drive?" "When?" The questions my family wanted answers were, "Is my wife / mom okay?"

Bragging Rights

IT is true that having a baby gave me bragging rights, but seriously, what does it really mean? Labor and Delivery Times: Oldest Son: 43.5 hours. Second Son: 23.5 hours. Third Son: 5.5 hours. I learned many things about having babies that helped me with stroke recovery. I was not concerned with time. I learned to trust myself, know I was not alone, and that I would be okay. I found that it was helpful to share some of the details with others. If possible, share your accomplishments with enthusiasm, a sense of adventure with those in your circle of family and friends so they can celebrate too.

It is true that regardless of the details of your child's birth, you have a beautiful little baby to show for it. Accomplishments after a stroke may not be as exciting, but for you and your supporters they feel pretty good.

Son #1, Andrew

LABOR: Contractions, but no progress. At 43.8 hours, the doctor wanted me moved from the birthing room to the delivery room. For the first time since I arrived at the hospital, the staff had something to do, other than ask me how I was feeling. The nurses moved me from a bed in the birthing room to a gurney and then to the delivery room. Someone moved me from the gurney to a different table in the delivery room. A nurse helped me get into position to birth this little baby. All of a sudden, the nurse told me, firmly, "Don't push!" The doctor asked, "What do you mean, 'don't push?'" No one knew that on my travels from the birthing room to delivery room, I was PUSHING. The doctor moved closer, saw that I had made progress. He said, "Now push." I did. And we met Andrew, Son #1 a few seconds later. That is what I do when nobody is looking.

Son #2, John

FOR the most part of our labor, we were left alone quite a bit of the time, which was helpful. I slept for five to ten minutes at a time, breathed through a sixty-second contraction and then back to my nap. When it was time to push, the doctor put one hand under the baby and delivered the baby one-handed. The doctor looked like he was catching a football. And that's how we met John, Son #2.

Son #3, Mark

WE were at Susan and Joe Lesser's Super Bowl party. At halftime, I got up to get some nachos and my water broke. Marcel and I went upstairs to call the doctor. When we turned around, everybody was standing there. Our two sons stayed with our dear friends, Melody and Mike Roe and there sons, Eric and Jared. We went to the hospital, watched the end of Super Bowl #23. San Francisco 49ers beat the Cincinnati Bengals 20-16. Joe Montana was the winning quarterback. Once the game was over, it was time to push and we met Mark, Son

#3.

Accomplishments and Excitement
1983, 1984, and 1989

I / we did it. We birthed our babies. Our family had three sons. Once I think about having the babies, the little ones growing up, they marry, and now our grandson is here, I start to cry tears of relief and tears of happiness every time.

September 1990

MY grandfather, Bill, who was 86 at the time, and his dear friend, 85-year-old Louise, had decided to marry. My husband and I and our three sons flew to Michigan to attend the wedding. It was important. They were darling. Did I mention that Marcel had to catch an earlier flight to get back to work, leaving me to fly back to Colorado with three boys by myself? An accomplishment is an accomplishment.

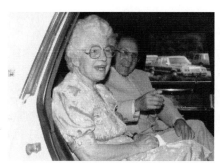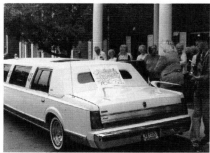

(Bill Davis and Louise Epperson, Wedding day,
September 15, 1990, Tonquish Creek Manor)

Brahms Lullaby

EVERY time a baby is born at St. Mary Mercy Hospital, "Brahms Lullaby" is played over the loud speaker throughout the hospital. When I was at work and I heard the Lullaby, my reaction was, "That is what happens at this hospital."

When I was a patient at the hospital after the stroke, hearing the Lullaby reminded me of all the families that I have met at the hospital, parents and little brothers and sisters waiting for another brother or sister. I observed babies being born. I met babies just hours after they were born—big babies, little babies, babies with lots of hair, bald babies, beautiful babies, and babies who needed a little extra care. I watched people becoming parents and parents becoming grandparents. Whenever I heard Brahms Lullaby on the hospital Public Address System, I thought, "They did it." Me, too.

September 2015

I drove to the library by myself. Ta Da! I love the library.

The Bestest News
May 2015

OUR family has had many good days and received happy news often. Several months after the stroke, we received the bestest news was that we were going to be grandparents. Our son, Andrew, and daughter-in-law, Justine, were expecting a baby. Happiness is everywhere. I couldn't have anticipated my grandson would become my personal therapist, trainer and buddy.

2015

Baby: Gestation, prenatal growth and development

Me: Recovery and Rest

Early 2016

Teddy: Born.

Grammy: Recovering.

Teddy Wednesdays: Music in the Park

We (Papa & Grammy): We gave Teddy time and our love; he knew he could depend on us. As our grandson started to stand, walk and talk, I followed his lead.

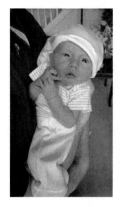 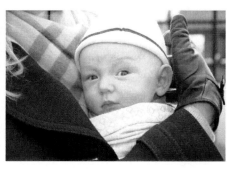

(Teddy. Permission to use granted by Andrew and Justine Madonna)

Fall 2016

Teddy: He spoke his first words and gave new names to Mimi, Daddy, Papa and Grammy. He smiled, laughed, crawled, stood up, sat down, and took first steps. He made his opinion known. He walked, ran, played, played, and played some more. He loved stories and long naps.

Grammy: My mobility improved, but still shaky. My speech continued to improve. I read and watched movies.

We: Teddy and I looked alike when we stood up from the floor. Bottoms up and then we grabbed something to hold on as we stood up. Teddy was trying everything: foods, moving, babbling, and exploring. I had not been able to do much a year ago, but taking baby steps. I am doing a little more. Teddy did not speak in complete sentences. It was up to us to figure out what he wanted; we paid attention. I did not always talk in complete sentences; I often used incorrect words; sometimes others would have to figure out what I wanted. It did not bother Teddy; he was cool. It did not bother me either. We shared many germs and colds.

Teddy's First Valentine's Day. Ever since the day we found out that Andrew and Justine were expecting a baby, we made a lot of plans, dreamed a lot of dreams. I drove to town, went in to one of my favorite stores, R.S.V.P. in downtown Plymouth and looked through all the Valentine Day cards until I found the perfect one for Teddy. While I was paying for it, I told the saleslady that it was for my first grandchild. The saleslady shared her "someday baby plans", baby names, and where she would live when she had a baby. I planned that trip to the card store for a long, long time. It was just as I had hoped and dreamed. "Happy First Valentine's Day, Teddy. Thank you, Mimi and Daddy for giving us this gift. You are great parents. "Happy Valentine's Day."

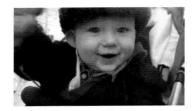

(Teddy. Permission to use granted by Andrew and Justine Madonna)

2017 & 2018

Teddy: Continued to meet all the developmental milestones. His words turned into sentences. Favorites: *Daniel the Tiger, Sesame Street, Boss Baby, Spy Kids*, riding his Thomas the Train. He picked dandelions for Grammy. Teddy was happy.

Grammy: Favorite: I loved Mr. Rogers. I returned to therapy as needed in between Teddy visits.

We: We were happy.

Teddy Wednesdays: We went to the library for story time, Barnes and Noble to play with Thomas the Train, and the apple orchard. We took field trips to Henry Ford Museum: visits with Santa Claus, snacks, big trains, old cars, Spirit of St. Louis. We went to Greenfield Village, rode all the rides: the train, Model T cars, horse drawn wagon, calliope, and Thomas the Train. Wednesdays was MiP (Music in the Park) concerts, Dairy King for ice cream, movies, and long naps. He always fell asleep on the way home from Henry Ford Museum and Greenfield Village; I was tired.

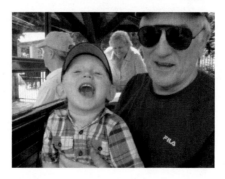

(Teddy and Papa. Permission to use granted by Andrew and Justine Madonna)

2019

Teddy: Teddy was a kid, growing and developing. Swim lessons, T-ball, soccer, and naps, sometimes and when needed. We had conversations about everything. Teddy was happy.

Grammy: My improvements kept pace with Teddy. I was able to speak in coherent sentences most of the time and if I was not tired.

We: We were happy. We walked around the house, careful to not fall down the groundhog holes.

Conversation: 9.4.19

> **Grammy:** "Teddy, this is how you do it."
>
> **Teddy:** "You're right, Grammy"

Conversation: 9.11.19

> I bumped into the train set and it came apart, Teddy said, "Silly Grammy."

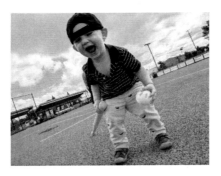

(This is Teddy. Permission to use granted by Andrew and Justine Madonna)

Bikes

Teddy: Teddy has a red bike with training wheels and it makes sounds.

Me: I have an adult-sized red Tricycle, with a horn and a basket.

We: Teddy and I are great biking partners. We ride around our driveway and throughout the neighborhood. One day, we met up with our neighbors, Lukas and Baylin, ages 6 and 7. Lukas drives an electric fire chief jeep. Teddy could not stop staring at the jeep. Lukas asked Teddy if he would like to ride with him in the jeep. Of course, Teddy nodded his head "yes." Lucas and Teddy went for a ride.

I think this was a developmental milestone for both of us: It was time for Teddy to make friends and ride off with them. It is time for Grammy to stand by and watch him go, with love and my blessings. I know it's a milestone because I have met this one before, watching my three sons go off with friends, old and new.

Next Year and Beyond

Teddy: Teddy should wear a tag that says, "Hi, I'm Teddy, and I am exploding with possibilities."

Grammy: Me, too.

We: We are happy. Papa and I are grateful to be a part of everything Teddy does. We are happy to be a part of this strong, kind, beautiful boy's life. Thank you, Andrew and Justine. Thank you, Teddy.

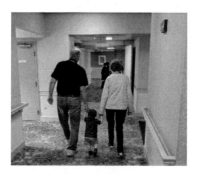

(Papa, Teddy and Grammy to visit Nonna. Permission to use granted by Andrew and Justine Madonna)

Year Three and Four Post stroke (PS). Healing in My Free Time

IN addition to taking medicine for high blood pressure, I have had positive experiences with walking, reiki , massage, exercising, swimming, bike riding, meditation, sound healing, music, reading, visualization, naps, daydreaming, manicures, spending time with family, friends and kitties, and spending time with myself. Oh yes, I almost forgot, visiting Paris.

If I had left the hospital, went home and sat, sat, sat all day long, my quality of life would have disintegrated. Instead, I adapted exercises to improve my balance, coordination and strengthening my core. There is not just one thing I did to magically make everything better, but if I chose nothing, the results would not be positive.

Having a stroke is not for the faint of heart. I spent a month in the hospital and rehabilitation, followed up with ongoing therapy, being willing to try new things, and having patience. Then, Poof! Five years goes by quickly, whoosh. How long will it take to get completely better? If I am lucky, I will improve forever.

Living in My Own World

I was living in La La Land for quite some time. I was so focused on what I had to do, I was not aware that others were living their lives, happy times, tough times, and sad times. Even when I became aware of the troubles others were experiencing, it was like watching a movie. It was not that I did not have empathy or understand what was happening, but knowing was not connected to my emotions. This is just one of the things that had to be reattached. Slowly I had to open the door and invite real people and real happenings into my brain and my thinking. Currently I respond appropriately and quickly to real troubles and good news with caring and I am willing to jump in to help. It was time for my helpers to return to their lives. I still live in La La Land part-time, leaving the window open for more happiness and joy.

"Our Grandson did the cutest thing." Everything Teddy does is cute. And he makes us happy. This Christmas, we bought an inflatable Santa and Snowman." It's what we needed. We needed to be happy. Now:

- I do not say, "I have a million things to do" because I do not have a million things to do anymore.

- If someone invites me to their house for dinner and tells me how hard they worked to make dinner, I will excuse myself, "So sad." If the host opens the door, her hair is not combed, and she is wearing her pajamas, I would say, "I am here, put me to work."

- My standard answer to getting out of a tricky situation: "Excuse me, I have a new book to read," or "Excuse me, I am going for a ride on my red trike."

Four Months Post Stroke (PS)

Walks

I walked with my friend, Lynne Hendzell. We walked outside, at the mall and inside at my old high school. We walked and walked about a mile or two or three, until I was tired. My friend, Lori Lee, suggested that we walk at Greenfield Village. We walked three to five miles, until I was tired. My friend, Diane Bogenrieder, took me shopping in Downtown Plymouth or to Newburg Lake. We walked until I was tired. Walking with Lynne, Lori and Diane got me out of the house. We had lots of therapeutic talking. After four years of walking and looking down so I would not trip, now I have to strengthen my core, stand up straight, swing both arms when I walk, and not drag my right foot... most of the time. The muscles in my right leg do not always remember to pick up my foot. Lori taught me how to tie my shoelaces with double bunny ears because my shoelaces are always untied.

Spring 2015, Grocery Shopping

WHEN we went grocery shopping, my husband went because we needed food. I went to see friends and make new friends. On that first trip to the grocery store, I held on to the grocery cart. The whole experience of making a list and getting the items on the list was lost on me. The shopping cart was my assistant. Under these circumstances, I didn't have to think, no asking what aisle is Frosted Flakes on. I didn't have to plan a menu and at this time, nothing tasted good. I certainly could not picture me running into a friend and chatting, but I did run into a friend on my first trip to Kroger. I ran into Michelle Dillon and we were happy to see each other. No questions, no thinking, but a place to walk, nothing has changed.

Fall 2015, Drive a Car

I drove to the library. Marcel was riding shotgun. He drove home because I was tired. A few weeks later, I drove to town and met my friends Michelle Dillon and Debbie Wardell for lunch at the Box Bar. I parallel parked perfectly. Now, it is time to get back on the road. Next stop, dinner with Mary Novrocki and Sally Welch, for one of our celebratory dinners that we have had since our children were in high school. We celebrate our children moving forward at these regularly scheduled dinners. This time, we will celebrate my steps forward, but I won't be driving, Sally will pick me up and we will meet Mary.

December 2015, Quilt Camp

MY friend, Gail Maloney, is a quilting artist; she took me with her to Quilt Camp in Chelsea, Michigan. There were 7 or 8 quilters at camp; we stayed in a beautiful house, quilts on every bed. The woman who owned the home made extremely delicious food. It was the first time I had been hungry in 11 months. I am not a quilter so I hung out in a comfy living room by myself. I read, listened to the ladies in the other room, and watched it snow all day. It was a religious experience.

August 2018, Mackinac Island

I wanted to ride a bike for a long time, but I did not think I would ever be able to ride a bike again. My balance was unsteady. I was not afraid of falling, but of breaking bones. On a trip to Mackinac Island, I rented a cute adult tricycle (trike). We pedaled around Mackinac Island, **8.2 miles. Ta Da!**

As soon as we got back from the trip, my husband and I both bought new bikes. Marcel chose a cool yellow bike and I decided on a sweet red trike with a basket. We live on the property where I grew up. Marcel and I rode to and from town, the same route I took when I was twelve years old. Some days, it felt like I pedaled fast and far enough, poof, I would be twelve again. As a twelve-year old, I rode my bike to town to my friend, Sherry's house and hung out. Now Marcel and I ride bikes to the library and Westborn Market, carrying groceries home in my basket. Just like when I was twelve, but I would have gone to Kemnitz Candy Store instead.

Twelve

When I was twelve, seventh grade, St. Peter's Lutheran Day School. I was free to go any place that I could ride my bike to. It was also the year I lost my mind over the Beatles. No more running around on recess. Sherry Hirth, Mary Berg, Sherry Siebert, Sue Ellen Sawusch, Judy Breitmeyer hung out talking about everything Beatles and making plans to go to the P&A Theater to see *A Hard Day's Night*.

I had a little incident last year, a fall, and no broken bones. A grape arbor's vines hanging over the sidewalk got tangled around my bike fender. I fell off the bike. My butt hit the ground first and then my helmet. The small scratches on my helmet could have been a big bump on my head. I heard the echo that the helmet made. Make a note: It was just an accident. I am okay. Make another note: Always wear a helmet when riding a bike. Helmets do not prevent accidents, but they do prevent booboos. All is well.

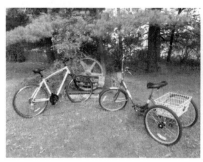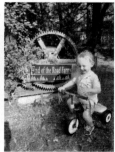

*(Teddy and our bikes. Permission to use granted by
Andrew and Justine Madonna)*

January 2019, Swimming

I swam as soon as I could walk. I loved the water, but I hadn't been swimming in a very long time. I do not know why. My friend, Barbra Well, asked me to go swimming with her at my old Plymouth High School pool. I hesitated because when I was in high school, the water was freezing. Eventually I said, "Sure." My body had forgotten how to swim and I was a little shaky. Geez, everything was brand new. The water was warm; it was heaven. I loved being in the water again. I moved freely. I exercised without tripping. I felt strong. I was free. I felt human instead of like a robot. I learned to swim once; I'll learn again.

Mr. Rogers swam almost every day.

September, 2019, Sioux Falls, South Dakota

I went to visit my friend, Marg Moxnes, in Sioux Falls, South Dakota all by myself. I flew in a big airplane. I was fretting about changing planes at Chicago O'Hare airport. I learned, once again, to put my fears out into the universe and someone will help you or offer "Special Assistance," a service of the airlines: transportation from the front door of the airport through TSA to the gate. It was successful. Oh, the most important thing, my dear friend and I had a happy time and I just knew it would be a great time. That is why I did something that terrified me and took that flight all by myself. Where should we go next, Marg?

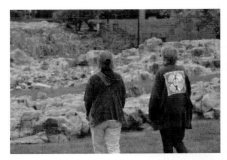
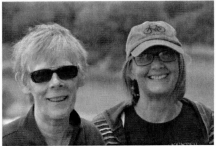
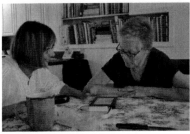

(Marg Moxnes and Deb, South Dakota and Michigan.
Permission to use granted by Marg Moxnes)

Greenhouses

ONE of my most favorite places to visit every winter is a greenhouse. My grand-parents had a greenhouse. C.W. built a tunnel from the house to the greenhouses, so that during the winter he didn't have to go outside. That may seem like a luxury, but do you know that to keep the greenhouse warm and the flowers safe, CW and Flora went out to the greenhouse every few hours at night to make sure the wood burning stove stayed hot. And during the summer, no matter how hot and humid it was in the greenhouse, the plants had to be watered all day long. The irrigation system had to be in good working order or crops could die in a short time.

The greenhouse and farm are long gone. The greenhouse and my grandpar-ents' house were taken by the State of Michigan and crushed when Interstate 275 was built. I hate Eminent Domain. I miss it all. I go to Matthaei Gardens at the University of Michigan, but my favorite place is Graye's Greenhouse, especially in the wintertime. When Mrs. Sylvia Graye passed away, I was so worried that would be the end of the greenhouse. I am so happy that Rachel Nisch bought it. I am so happy to see how Rachel and Jessica Anchor are doing so many cool things. It reminds me of my grandparents' greenhouse, the warmth in the winter, the smell of the plants. It feels like home.

Five Years Post Stroke (PS), Crossing the Street

HOW old were you when you crossed the road by yourself…safely? Every time you crossed the road? I was always very responsible, followed all the rules. After the stroke, crossing the road became a challenge. As soon as the sign displayed, "Walk". I started to cross the street, but speed was not my friend. I only got half way and the sign flashed."Stop?""Go Back?" I now walk faster and cross the street in a timely fashion.

The dilemma I had then and still do, five years later, standing at the crosswalk, seeing the traffic light and the walk signs at the same time. I have to think for a moment, "What?" This does not happen when I drive; everything is automatic. But when I walk or ride my bike, I often wait for two or three light changes. So, from a lady, I will gladly accept your help when I cross the street.

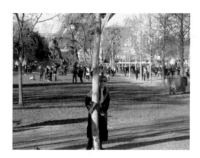

(Deb, Paris)

Everything works, but not the same as before

DURING the past five years, my world moved in slow motion. The changes have been subtle, others dramatic and confusing. There has been more progress than setbacks. I do not wish for all the old me to come back and get rid of all that I have been given. That is preposterous. Life does not work like that. I cannot change what has happened, but I can make changes going forward. I could say I cannot believe all that has happened, but it is not true. I can believe it. I embrace it all. I love what I had. I love what I have now.

I am not complaining, just observing to help me understand what has happened and what is next. Not every moment is good and not every moment is bad. It is my responsible to make sure I grab all the good days, happiness, giggles, and joy. I hesitate to jump for joy because I think you may understand, I am not always steady and jumping makes me a little nervous.

Five years ago, I could not stand alone, walk or talk at all. I have not always been able to stand alone and I could not walk at all. Slowly, I have moved with less assistance. All that I could not do five years ago, I have regained abilities. It took awhile to be able to move without assistance and now I can move alone. Standing tall, my hands on my hips, I can move everything. Today, I move through life vertically with ease and grace. I am grateful that my cognition and memory are intact. My helpers stand by my side and do not have to hold me up. My hands up in the air. Ta Da. I am happy.

Thoughts

After

After I survived the accident in my brain
and it was time to go home,
I was a bit lost.
Would I recognize my house?
The real test of what I remember would be confirmed
when I walked through the back door.

Months before I had the stroke, I was determined,
obsessed to put my neglected
pictures and frames on all of the walls,
which had been abandoned
and kept in a room in the back of the house.
I gathered all the pictures and my hammer.
The "tap-tap-tap-tap-tap"
signaled another picture had found their spot on the wall.
Tap-tap-tap-tap-darn-tap-tap-darn-darn
never discouraged me.
There was no stopping until every picture was in its very own place.
Finally, all the walls were covered
with photographs and embroidered artworks.
Everything in the house was where it was supposed to be.

It would be more than another two weeks before I could go up the stairs.
to the second floor,
to the walls that held my children's pictures,
all the faces I loved.
I would never be lonely or afraid again.

p.s. If you have a chance to see "The Picture Wall of Boys", but crooked pictures make you nervous, then step away, go away. Nothing and no one is perfect.

CHAPTER 9

THE POWER OF MY FAMILY

IT is hard to tell my family how I appreciated everything they did for me. I know what they did and I wanted them to know that I knew. I had the stroke, but the whole family was affected, everyone in a different way. There were scary times for them, but they always had strength enough to stand by my side. Under normal circumstances, I would be doing everything, asking everyone lots of questions, and gathering all the relevant information to make things better. I was part of the decision-making team, but not this time. Being the focus is not my comfort zone.

My family told me I was okay; I believed them. My family noticed even the smallest of improvements I made each day and I believed them. I did not ask my family many questions. It's only been in the last year that I wanted to ask my family questions about their view of "the stroke."

- Who notified Marcel that I was in the hospital?
- Who found my car?
- When did you get to the hospital?
- During the first 48 hours, how long did you stay at the hospital?
- What did you think?
- How were you?

Marcel

I do not know all that my husband did while I was in the hospital, but I know that he did everything and whatever needed to be done. He answered all the medical staffs' questions, discussed treatment plans and discharge plans. He was available every day. Marcel answered phone calls, emails and texts. He heard all the news first, and then he shared it with our children. During the first days in the hospital, the news was uncertain. There was no indication that I would walk, be able to take care of myself, or wake up. He had to share that news with our children, as well. My family waited.

February 8, 2015. Marcel posted this note on facebook, "I am sorry I haven't been able to post something sooner, but you can imagine that things have been very difficult for the past couple of weeks. I'd like to thank everyone for their prayers, their support, and their good wishes. I can't tell you how much that means to me and to Deb. I'm sure most of you know that she suffered a hemorrhagic stroke on the 27th of January. I am very happy to say that she is doing extraordinarily well and we expect her to make a full recovery. It will take time and we'll need a lot of support, but she is improving every day. She is walking a little bit and her speech is coming along nicely. Please keep those prayers coming in our direction. They are working."

When Marcel and I started dating, I came down with the flu. I was really sick. He drove from Detroit after working all day, taking classes at Wayne State at night, and brought me Chinese food. It worked. I felt better. What I can say about my husband is that I learned when he can help, he does; when he needs help, he accepts it. We are there for each other. That is a big deal. When I run into a rough patch, I often have a craving for Chinese food.

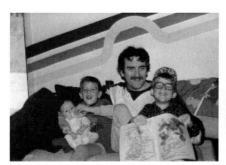 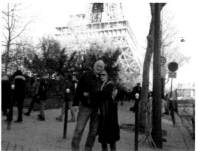

(Mark, Andrew, Marcel and John)

Home Movies

I especially like videos of people who have faced challenges, been down, and eventually got up. They persevere. They crawl across a finish line. I love those videos. There is a video of a little elephant, lying on his back in a mud pit. He could not get up. His mother and the other elephants tried to get him out with no success. Lions surrounded them. It was so scary. The elephants pulled the mother away from the little elephant. An old female elephant stayed behind. It took a while, but she freed the baby from the pit. Yes, I love that video.

I told my husband, "Darn it. I wish someone had taken pictures or videos of me on the first day of therapy, the following weeks, months, up until today. I would have liked to see "the progress."

My husband said, "I did take your picture. You didn't like it."

"No, not that picture," I said. It was a picture of me the first week that I was in the hospital, lying in bed, ill, no makeup, not groomed at all.

I wanted a picture of the progress I made.

My husband wanted me to get better, to be well.

All My Children

A promise: treat my sons according to their ages, but I am allowed to remember and reminisce about them at any age, anytime, look at old pictures, and send them a copy. The three sons that I gave birth to years ago are the same three sons that were at my bedside when I woke up January 29, 2015. And they are still here.

Andrew, Justine, and Teddy

ANDREW and Justine became loving parents 4 years ago. Five years ago, they stood by my side, asked how I was feeling, listened to what I said, never correcting me.

April 5, 2015. We all went out to brunch on Easter Sunday. I used a walker; I did not feel dressed up; my taste buds were still off; and I was not hungry. My table manners were adequate, still a little messy, but this lunch was the best I'd had in a long time. We were together.

When I found out I was going to be a grandmother, I wanted to be called, "Happy." I wanted to have a big grin on my face because all babies deserve their

Grandmother's smiles. Just before the baby was born, I told Justine I wanted my smile back. Even after a very long labor, Justine said, "You still have the smile." I was relieved.

Andrew and Justine's little baby was born at St. Joseph Hospital, the same hospital that Andrew was born in. We met Teddy about an hour after he was born. Andrew handed Teddy to me. Teddy was born and Andrew laid him in my arms, lots of happiness. When Teddy was four and a half months, he began staying with Papa and Grammy on Wednesdays. Even if my smiles were subdued, happiness is always there. What a treat to be a part of my son's life as a father to my grandson.

1983: I became a C.O.T.A. (Certified Occupational Therapist Assistant, Schoolcraft College). I thought that having a baby while I was going to school would be okay. We were moving out of state to Arvada, Colorado. I had to finish my program in Michigan first. *(Advice to self: next time, go to college as soon as you are out of high school.)*

My classmates threw a baby shower for me and Andrew on the lawn outside our classroom. I returned to school when Andrew was 3 weeks old. I took my certification test when Andrew was 5 months old. I do not know how I did it because I certainly had "new mom fog". I carried Andrew, at 5 months old, across the stage to receive my diploma. We did it.

When Andrew was younger, he gave me a coffee can covered with pink construction paper for Mother's Day: "the one and only Happy Mother's Day Coupon Can". The instructions were on the top of the can, "These coupons are good for life. We must stop what we're doing to do it". Inside the coffee can were 44 coupons: "Do any chore." "Make dinner." "Clean my room." "Help Mark with his homework." "Free Hugs." "Anything."

I wish I had not been so foolish to ask my children to do chores. I should have asked them what they would like to do to help around the house because they are part of a family or I could have pulled a coupon from the perfect Mother's Day gift.

When Andrew and Justine married, their florist asked my name, and then she gave me a wrist corsage. My flower arrangement was just a little different from the rest. My corsage had an iris. I had once told Justine that I loved wild blue irises. The iris in my yard was planted by my grandmother, Flora, 40 years ago. The irises return each spring.

Justine is a loving mom, even tempered. It has been fun watching her with Teddy. I have learned so much from Justine observing her and Teddy. She gets down and close to Teddy; whatever she says to him is between the two of them. Justine is so wise and kind; I want to be her. Becoming a grandmother, Grammy, to a little boy who has such loving parents is a joy. Teddy loves his parents. Andrew and Justine love Teddy. I love my grandson. I love my children.

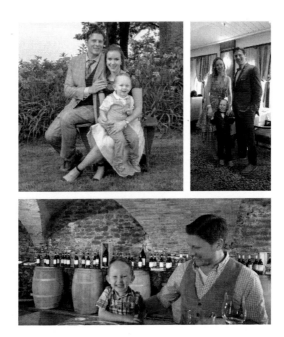

(Andrew, Justine, and Teddy.
Permission to use granted by Andrew and Justine Madonna)

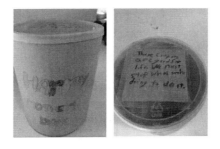

(The Wise Coffee Can)

John and Rebecca

JOHN lived in Chicago for several years. It was his idea that we visit different ball parks around the country: Pittsburgh, Cleveland, and Baltimore. He and Mark made it to Fenway Park. I am still sad about missing that one.

John is a high school Math teacher and a musician. He traveled back and forth while I was in the hospital. Before school started, the students hung out in the cafeteria. One morning, John, the teacher / musician, told the students that his mom was in the hospital. He played the guitar and sang "All You Need Is Love"; the students joined in. John told them that it would mean a lot to me. He did not just tell me about it, he showed me the video. He was correct and even though I was still muddled, I felt like my old self for a few minutes.

Depression, panic attacks, and crying kicked in a few weeks after I came home from the hospital. John continued to come home on weekends. We binged on *The West Wing* and *Lost*. When it was time for him to get to the train, I wept and could not stop. I never ever cried like that. I knew that must have made him feel horrible.

December 2016, John introduced us to Rebecca. It was always a treat to have them visit. They cooked for us, lots of vegetables. It has only taken us a couple years to eat more and more vegetables. And I never ever, ever thought I would eat Brussels sprouts and think they were delicious. I never thought I would say I like vegetables, but I do, "Sam I am." We want John and Rebecca to know that we listened to them.

One beautiful day, I do not really remember if the day was sunny or cloudy, warm or cold, but one really nice day, we received a note from John and Rebecca. They asked us if we would like to go to Paris with them, mais bien sûr. They gave me a journal and asked us to give them a list of things we would like to see and do while in Paris. I was a little nervous because I was concerned about how I would navigate in a new place.

A few months before going to Paris, John and Rebecca came home. We talked about all that we would do in Paris. John and Rebecca suggested we pick up a few books about Paris. I left the room for a few minutes, returning with an armload of books about Paris, but not all my Paris books. Rebecca tapped John on the shoulder. "What?" I asked. Rebecca said that John just wanted me to be happy. Happy about going with them to Paris? Je suis très heureux.

John and Rebecca compiled an itinerary, wish list, and found an Airbnb, 2 bedrooms, 2 baths. We spent two weeks in Paris, staying only a few blocks from Rue Mouffetard, a street filled with restaurants and markets. We went to a bakery every morning to buy a croissant. I was an appreciative tourist and I loved everything. We spent the last few days staying a block from the Arc de'Triomphe and walking on the Champs-Élysées on a "no drive Sunday."

Months before John and Rebecca asked us to go to Paris, Rebecca and I spoke about travelling. John and Rebecca love to travel. I told her that I didn't think I would be travelling very much, maybe a trip to Northern Michigan. I told her that the only place I ever wanted to visit was Paris. After we returned home from Paris, I again told John and Rebecca that I was so excited and I could not believe that I got to see and do everything I wanted. When John and I were alone, John said that Rebecca planned the trip for me. I love Paris. I love my children.

This is my # 1 favorite memory of Paris. We walked along the Seine. Notre Dame to the left and Shakespeare and Company to the right. We walked behind John and Rebecca, who were in love and I held my husband's hand.

#2 Memory. Musee D'Orsay.

#3 Memory. Jardin des Plantes.

#4 Memory. Holding hands walking along the Seine.

#5 Memory. We went into a French bookstore. All the books were in French and everyone spoke French, but I did not have to speak French to enjoy the atmosphere. I asked, "Où est Le Petit Prince?" I was so proud, but when they told me where it was in French, je n'ai pas compris. The kind bookseller said, "Follow me"; he handed me a copy of *Le Petit Prince*. I said, "Merci," of course. I sat down with the book and I found the words I understood and I looked at the pictures. J'etais si herueux. *The Little Prince* in English or French is one of my favorite stories. We also visited The Little Prince store (TLP) and I bought several TLP treasures.

#6 Memory. Pack light.

#7 Memory. Special thanks to friends who sent me tips and texts about what to do while we were in Paris: Gail Maloney, Anya Linda Dely Dietz, and Diane Bogenrieder,

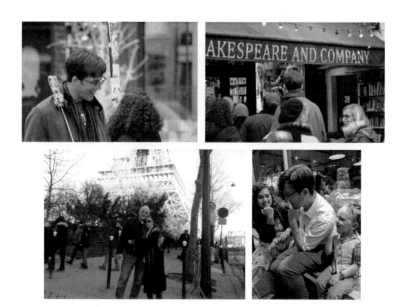

*(John, Rebecca, Marcel and Deb, Paris. John, Rebecca and Teddy, Seattle.
Permission to use granted by Andrew and Justine Madonna,
John Madonna and Rebecca Mitrovich)*

Mark and Amanda

MARK told me he understood the seriousness of the stroke, but he knew I would get better. If you think that is a simple way to look at things, you are wrong. There is nothing more powerful that to have someone be convinced that you are going to be all right.

On the first day of kindergarten, I picked Mark up from school. I asked, "How was your first day of kindergarten? What did you do?" This little boy looked up at me and said, "Do we have to talk about it? I was there all day". My response, "What time can we talk about it?" Mark gave me a time that we can discuss what goes on with school. It took me a few days to get the message. He did what he was supposed to do; after school was his time. He did say it was okay to take him to and from school, just do not ask so many questions.

I was fixated on knowing every detail of Mark's day, I observed the children at school, moving, and playing. I learned much about children and how they interacted with the world around them. I learned from Jane Goodall, who learned about chimps by watching them and not asking them how their day was or ask why they did what they did. It was simple. he told what I needed to know. It was all okay.

A lesson that took me forever to learn is that when I told Mark to hurry up, he went the same speed as when I did not tell him to hurry up. As I stepped back and observed his brothers and my husband, they, too, went the same speed when I told them to hurry up as they did when I did not say anything. This is my apology: "I am very sorry for telling you to hurry up."

In 2008, I participated in the Susan G. Komen 3-Day 60 mile walk to raise funds to fight for a cure for breast cancer and promote on the "Hearts for Gretchen" team in honor of Gretchen, Suzie, Johanna and Heidi's sister. The team: Suzie Pitluk, Gretchen Pitluk (Suzie's daughter), Nathan Pitluk (Suzie's son), Eric Surprenant, Elena Surprenant, Linda Brunetto, and Jack Pitluk (our team's wingman).

At the final stop of the third day, I sent a text to my family that I had 3 miles to go. Mark sent me a text back: "Keep walking."

Mark loves baseball. From the time he could read, he learned everything about baseball, the players, and the statistics. When he played Little League baseball, he was the guy who knew everything about baseball. We watched the Ken Burns' documentary, *Baseball*, before we went to Cooperstown. On our trip to and from the Baseball Hall of Fame, we listened to audio books and videos about baseball. I like the stories, the drama of baseball: *The Green Fields of the Mind* by A. Bartlett Giamatti; *Hub Fans Bid Kid Adieu* by John Updike; Game 6, 1975, Carlton Fisk, waving the ball fair, Boston Red Sox; Game 1, October 15, 1988, Kurt Gibson's home run, Los Angeles Dodgers; all Detroit Tigers, *Field of Dreams;* and anything about Ted Williams.

Ten years after our trip to Cooperstown, Mark became a part of the Miracle League of Plymouth, a baseball league for special needs children, when the field was only a dream. He is now a MLP board member, the coach of the Yellow Jackets team, a buddy on the field, umpire, catcher, and everything else.

His knowledge of baseball came in handy for a benefit for the Miracle League of Plymouth players, families and volunteers: "The Perfect Game." On a Thursday night in February, 2013, at the Mayflower Meeting House in Plymouth, alumni from the Detroit Tigers World Series Championship teams of 1968 and 1984 told stories about the attributes of those outstanding Tiger teams and their exploits on the baseball field.

Detroit Tigers 1968 Alumni: Hal Naragon (coach), Mickey Stanley, Tom Matchick, Gates Brown and Denny McLain.

Detroit Tigers 1984 Alumni: Dave Bergman, Dave Rozema, Barbaro Garbey and Dan Petry.

Emcee: Eli Zaret

Mark coordinated with the company, WhatIfSports.com, to simulate who would win between the 1968 Detroit Tigers and the 1984 Detroit Tigers. To determine this, there were 101 7-game series simulated between the two teams. The 1968 Tigers were victorious in 67 of the 101 series.

1968 versus1984 Detroit Tigers

	Series Wins	%	4-Game Series Wins	%	5-Game Series Wins	%	6-Game Series Wins	%	7-Game Series Wins	%
1968 Tigers	67	66.3%	11	10.9%	16	15.8%	20	19.8%	20	19.8%
1984 Tigers	34	33.7%	4	4.0%	6	5.9%	12	11.9%	12	11.9%
Total	101	100.0%	15	14.9%	22	21.8%	32	31.7%	32	31.7%

(Permission to use granted by Mark Madonna)

Last year, Mark introduced us to Amanda or, as Teddy calls her, "Aunt Panda." I taught Amanda how to make crepes. Amanda's crepes were more attractive than mine. Both of our crepes were delicious, but Amanda's were more authentic, very French. and they were delicious. I have realized that I have a lot to learn from Amanda. It is always nice to have a team making meals. Amanda and Mark took charge of the Christmas cookie baking with Teddy. Amanda and Mark gave us a gift certificate for cooking class at Sur La Table for a Christmas present so we could learn to make croissants. It was fun. There were plenty of delicious croissants for the four of us to take home. Amanda and Mark know that if you are not going to Paris, croissants are the next best thing.

Amanda is an opera singer. Her gift to me is she brought classical music back into my life. She has recommended songs I might like: Leonard Bernstein's *Candide*; I forgot how much I love it; "Make Our Garden Grow" has always been one of my favorite songs. Amanda's voice range is Coloratura Soprano like Beverly Sills. I have always loved Beverly Sills. Amanda introduced me to "The Willow Song", sung by Beverly Sills, from *The Ballad of Baby Doe*, which I had never heard before; it made me cry, It was so beautiful. Giving me music that I used to love has been a blessing. I have been searching and you-tubing operas. I discovered the opera, *The Little Prince* by Rachel Portman. I had never heard it before. I cannot stop listening to it. In my imagination, I see and hear Amanda, singing in our yard one day. I do.

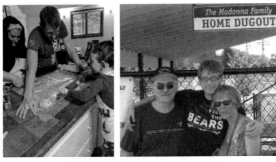

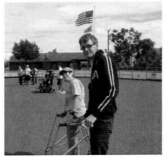

(Amanda, Mark and Teddy. Making Cookies. Marcel, Mark and Deb, Miracle League of Plymouth, the Bilkie Family Field. Jamie Jones and Mark, MLP, Permission to use granted by Susan and Jamie Jones, Mark Madonna and Amanda Xydis, Andrew and Justine Madonna)

Dear Andrew, Justine, Teddy, John, Rebecca, Mark, and Amanda

THANK you for being you, for being in our life. You are all a blessing. You have done things that touch my heart. Thank you for my favorite gift, serendipity.

Little Anecdotes about My Family

THESE little tales have nothing to do with having a stroke or recovery, but I thought about them when I was in the hospital and home recovering. This is our family. These stories belong here.

#1. The Rock and Independence Day

WE planned a road trip, traveling to Denver, New Mexico, Houston, Graceland, and home again. We purchased a conversion van: comfy chairs and a video player. Yes, there was only one video player for five people. That does not sound too fancy now, but it was nice. We packed everything we needed for a three-week cross country trip.

Marcel drove the first shift. I chose the first movie, *Mr. Holland's Opus*. I love that movie. This movie always makes me cry, but I cry alone. That was the only time any of my movies were played on this trip. Next movie, *The Rock*. Next movie, *Independence Day*. Next, *The Rock*. Next, *Independence Day*, etc. There were other choices, but those two movies were the only ones viewed and enjoyed for the next three weeks. Boys - 4 vs. Girl - 1

I wanted to go to Graceland. No one else wanted to go to Graceland. I promised we would stop just long enough so that we could have our Christmas picture taken in front of Graceland. About an hour before we arrived in Memphis, we had a flat tire. No Graceland. No pictures.

I thought of this when I was in a hospital room with everyone there. I fondly remember being in a van with my family and watching Mr. Holland's Opus. We could have also watched The Rock and Independence Day while I was in the rehab unit for three weeks. That would have been perfect.

#2. Where are the Tricorders?

I have watched Star Trek since it debuted in 1966. My family watched every version of Star Trek: The Original, Next Generation, Deep Space Nine, Voyager, etc. So I wanted to know why Bones McCoy had a Tricorder and my doctors did not have one. I was sure my doctors wanted one, too. I cannot have an MRI because I have metal in my leg. The Tricorder would be useful. My son, John, pointed out that the original Captain Kirk's Star Trek took place in the year 2265. So next, I suppose no one can beam me up either.

#3. Ernie Harwell

WHEN Andrew and John were six and eight, they played Little League Baseball. They loved baseball, baseball cards, and the Detroit Tigers. At one of the baseball games, hats were handed out to the children. Sitting at a baseball game, I closed my eyes, and imagined what it is like for a child walking into a stadium for the first time. I keep those memories of those who loved baseball. My grandmother, Blanche, loved listening to baseball on the radio, not television.

Ernie Harwell, the beloved announcer for the Detroit Tigers, was scheduled to make an appearance at a store in Plymouth. Someone had painted a picture of Ernie and he would autograph the paintings. Andrew, John and I went downtown to see if we could meet Ernie. They wore their Little League hats and shirts. I still regret that Mark, age two, and Marcel did not go with us.

When we arrived at the store, I asked the sales lady if my sons could meet Ernie. The lady walked to the back of the store where Ernie was sitting. Andrew and John didn't their eyes off Ernie. The lady returned and whispered to me, "What are their names?" I told her. She left again and talked to Ernie. The lady waved to us, to come on back. Halfway to Ernie, standing, with his magical voice, "Andrew, John, I have been waiting for you". Ernie bent down, shook their hands, "Where have you been?" Andrew and John answered together, "My mom was making dinner."

Ernie asked them how their teams, calling their teams by name, were doing. Ernie asked Andrew and John if he could sign something for them. They had brought the hats they had received at the Tigers game. When Ernie handed the hats back, Andrew reached behind him, grabbing the third hat he had in his back pocket. "Could you sign this hat, too? It is for my brother, Mark? He is only two years old; he is home with our dad." Ernie asked them to tell Mark and their dad he was sorry he did not meet them. "Boys, thank you for stopping by."

When we got home, Andrew and John told Mark and their dad about Ernie. Andrew handed Mark his hat. The boys loved meeting Ernie and so did I. I took notes on how Ernie interacted with my two sons and including the son at home. I thought it would come in handy someday. I wanted to be just like Ernie when I grew up.

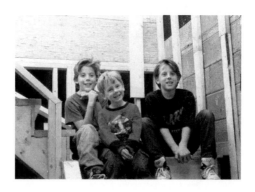

(John, Mark, and Andrew, building a house)

#4. Flora and Loretta

OUR cats, Flora and Loretta, are very different. Flora, whether I was well or ill, needed her humans to take care of her, provide food, unending affection, and pet her forever. When I returned home from the hospital, Loretta slept on my right arm and did that for many more nights. They took care of me and I took care of them. That is how we protect each other.

In the movie, "Alien," Ripley, the main character, was the last survivor on a ship travelling through space. Her fellow crew members had been killed one by one by an alien. The ending was scary and Ripley battled with the alien. Just when we thought Ripley was safe, she discovered that Jonesy, the cat, is somewhere in the ship. Despite the danger, Ripley searches for Jonesy. Ripley finds Jonesy and carries her to the safety of the shuttle. Ripley locks the door, but, unknown to her, the alien was also in the shuttle. I do not remember all the details because the alien was gross. Ripley finally destroyed the alien and she prepared to go back to earth. Ripley held Jonesy in her lap. That is how a woman and a cat protect each other.

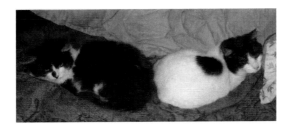

(Flora and Loretta, named after my grandmother and godmother)

p.s.

Dear Sons,

I am sorry for all the endless times I told you to "Hurry Up".

Dear Daughters,

Trust me, don't tell my sons to "Hurry Up". It does not work.

Dear Grandson,

Do not grow up too quickly. Take your time.

Dear Husband,

Thank you for tying my shoes. Thank you for working all day, go to classes at night, and then bring me Chinese food when I was not feeling so well.

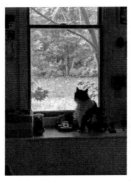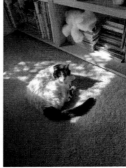

(Flora and Loretta)

Thoughts

Safe at Home

slide home
    walk home
        walk-off home run
            tagged at home
come home with me
my home is your home
    second home
        home away from home
            room at our house
                home-cooked meal
                    it feels like home
        I can see home with my eyes closed
going home
    stay home
        home is sweet
    home

CHAPTER 10

The Power of Others

MANY of the books and movies I enjoyed when I was a young reader had a thread running through them: Lassie, *The Little Princess*, *Pollyanna*, and *Captain January*. I read *Heidi* when I was 7 or 8 and watched the Shirley Temple movie over and over. Heidi had a Grandfather. I had a Grandfather. Heidi lived with her Grandfather on the mountains. I lived with my Grandfather on a farm. Heidi helped her friend, Clara, walk again. I believed I could help others to walk again. I wanted to help people walk, run, or do anything. Lassie helped everyone and there were times that Lassie needed help, too.

From fictional characters to real-life people, I could see how powerful they were, even in their struggles. I just wanted to know everything they were dealing with: Helen Keller, Anne Frank, and Franklin Roosevelt. Harold Russell was a returning veteran, a double amputee, both arms below the elbow, who portrayed a veteran, a double amputee in a wonderful movie, *The Best Years of Our Lives*.

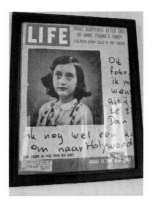

(LIFE Magazine, August 18, 1958, one of many 1950s and 1960 LIFE Magazines that C. W. Good read and saved and I inherited.)

When I heard about someone's illness or condition, I never thought I had "the disease". I was curious and I always wanted to learn more. As I grew up, I expanded my "medical practice" to diagnosing conditions and creating treatment plans for others. I did not charge for this information because I kept it to myself. This "imaginary medical practice" I have came in handy when I dealt with my illness in a logical, practical, and creative way.

Jamie Jones
It's a Good Day to Have a Good Day

I met Jamie when she was 10 years old at "Music in the Park", (MiP). She has been at every summer Wednesday concert from the beginning. She attends every Thursday night concert, Friday night concert, and "Art in the Park". She goes to the library every Saturday. She takes art classes, yoga, and bowling. Jamie loves being out about town and running into people she knows. Even if she does not know you, she will love you. She loves jewelry and is always wearing a lot of bling, even when she plays Miracle League baseball (MLP). She loves music and when the "Star Spangled Banner" is played, she weeps.

At a MiP concert, when the music starts, she is so happy. If the performers give a shout out to Jamie from the stage, she squeals. S-Q-U-E-A-L-S. A squeal is prolonged sharp cry of surprise, not a screech or scream or a shriek or squawk or a howl. It is Happiness.

Last year, Jamie's mother, Susan, and our dear friend, Beverly, (Beverly Meyer, "The Music Lady" performs at Music in the Park), threw "a Surprise Squeal Party" for Jamie with surprises, food and music. I entered the house first. Jamie is always happy to see me, of course; but when she saw Beverly, she clapped and, cheered, and squealed. With all the excitement, Jamie became quiet, taking it all in. Everyone but Jamie ate lunch. After lunch, there was music and singing. Jamie sat on the floor in front of Beverly, an audience of one. Beverly sang. Susan and I were the roadies. It was the *Bestest Day Ever*.

A few months ago, Beverly, Susan and I decided it was time for another "Bestest Day Ever Surprise Squeal Party" for Jamie. My grandson, Teddy, Stella (Jamie's niece), Gavin (Jamie's nephew), and Dave (Jamie's dad) were part of the surprise this year. I explained to Teddy that we were going to go to a Squeal Party. I explained that meant Jamie was happy, really happy. From now on, I don't think

Teddy will believe anyone who says they are happy if they're not squealing. We all had another Bestest Day Ever. A third "Squeal Party" is in the planning stage.

How many people do you know explode with happiness?

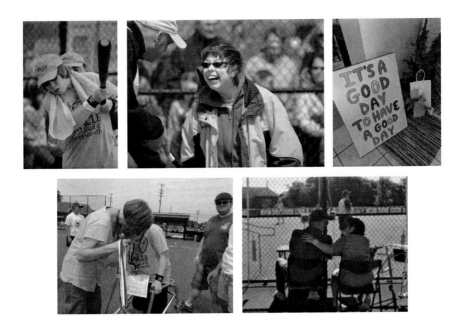

(*Jamie Jones, Marcel, and Deb, Miracle League of Plymouth. A gift from Jamie Jones. Permission to use granted by Susan and Jones and Mark Madonna*)

Alex Ham-Kucharski
Diagnosis

ALEX'S mom and dad, Dawn and Rich Ham-Kucharski, and I are always amazed when people say that Alex "will never do this or that." We love it because if we received $100 every time someone said it, we would have lot of money. Double that if they did not have a license for that crystal ball they pretend to use to pre-determine Alex's future.

Alex is a real person and my friend. I have known Alex since he was 3 years old. Now he's 22 years old. Alex graduated from high school in Georgia in 2016. On a trip to Michigan, he stopped in to see me, wearing his cap and gown. He knew his graduation was important to me. Ta Da, Alex. I have watched him grow up. He survived middle school in four different states: Texas, New Jersey, Michigan, Georgia. My reason for telling you about Alex is that he is a remarkable young man, and he has accomplished things I could only dream that he would do. I have been a witness to his successes and his battles. I look forward to the "nexts" for Alex.

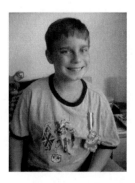

(Alex and Courage. Permission to use granted by Alex Ham-Kucharski and Dawn Ham-Kucharski)

Medical Diagnosis. I will start with the Perinatal Stroke that Alex experienced an hour before birth. Alex's official diagnosis, per his mother, Dawn, is Alexisms.

- Profound Sensor neural Hearing Loss
- Large Vestibular Aqueduct Syndrome
- Auditory Processing Disorder
- Expressive speech delay
- Cerebral Palsy
- Autism, a Developmental Neurological Disorder
- Chronic Migraines
- Sixth Spinal Lumbar
- Torticollis
- Duplicate 8P23 Genetic Disorder
- GJB3 Genetic Disorder

- Duplicate Superior Vena Cava emptying into his Coronary Sinus and flooding it and a Brindle Blockage
- NASH, non-alcoholic steatohepatitis
- Severe GERD
- Precancerous Colon Polyps
- Precancerous Moles
- Depression
- Anxiety
- Bone Marrow Blood Disorder

College

Alex is in year four of college. After all, he graduated from high school; the logical next step was college.

- Georgia Gwinnett College in Lawrenceville, Georgia.
- Major in political science. Minor in religious studies.
- He has applied to transfer to University of North GA into the East Asian Studies program with a concentration in Japan.
- During the summer of 2018, Alex studied abroad, three weeks of six credit hours, plus other activities at Otemon Gaukin University in Osaka Japan, along with two weeks in Myajima, Kyoto, Hiroshima, Tokyo, and Kamakura Japan. An earthquake had occurred in Japan shortly before Alex arrived in Japan.

And:

- Four years recipient of the Quota International of Northside Atlanta John T. Wheeler Scholarship
- Four Years Recipient of The Hope Scholarship of Georgia
- Dean's List Recipient 2017, 2018, 2019
- Golden Key National Honor Society 2019-present

What's next for Alex? You wouldn't believe it. Alex will tell you in his book.

Fun

ALEX was my advisor when the Miracle League of Plymouth was created. Alex had played Miracle League Baseball in Frisco, Texas, and he knew what it was all about. Currently he plays Miracle League Baseball in Cumming, Georgia

and:

Special Olympics: Track and Field, Bowling, Swimming, Power Lifting, Equestrian.

and:

Alex takes private equestrian lessons.

and

Alex sponsors a one-eyed 16-year-old rescue horse named, Lenape.

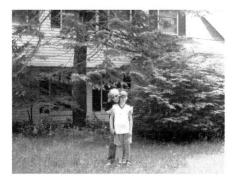

(This photo was taken in my front yard in 2009,
6 years before my stroke and 11 years after

Alex's Perinatal Stroke. Permission to use granted by Alex Ham-Kucharski and Dawn Ham-Kucharski)

Alex & I are Friends and Stroke Survivors.

One had a stroke.

One will have a stroke.

His stroke took place (in utero) at 4 p.m., June 26, 1998.

He was born at 5:02 pm., June 26, 1998.

A Brain Bleed, affecting White Matter & Lower Left Temporal Lobe.

My stroke will take place January 27, 2015

at 63 years old.

Left-Side Hemorrhagic Stroke, (a bleed), in the Basal Ganglia.

Strokes affected both.

They experienced many changes

But some things never change.

Alex & I are still friends

We are both perfect.

Sandy Sagear
Imagine ... Sandra Sagear did

POLIO was a dreaded disease and it still exists. Efforts to rid the world of Polio continue. It affected adults, and children, and the man who would become the President of the United States, Franklin Delano Roosevelt. Names for Polio included Infantile Paralysis and Paralytic Polio. Sandy acquired Polio before a vaccine was developed; she contracted polio when she was seventeen months old.

Sandy attended a three-story high school with no elevator, (1966 -1969). The Americans with Disabilities Act, (ADA), would not be enacted until 1991. This was typical of multi-storied building built in the early 20th century. The building was not retrofitted with elevators for years. The school administration did not encourage her to attend this school. Sandy wanted to go to school, this school, with friends, with all the other kids. Sandy wore metal braces which made walking up and down stairs ill-advised and unsafe. She used a back staircase to get to the second floor. She scooted up the stairs on her bottom to the second floor, wearing a skirt. She did not have a backpack. Friends carried her books up and down the stairs, but not every day. All her classes were on the second floor, the second floor library was her lunchroom too. She accepted the challenge because she wanted to go to school. And she did graduate with the Plymouth High School Class (PHS) of '69. She had a great family, friends and she was one predetermined young woman with a kind heart. I was one of her friends.

"Can't never did anything. *Can* did it all." —Sandy Sagear

*The Sandra Sagear Wall of Courage at the new Plymouth High School
by Vonnie Bench, Josh Bench, Tiffany Lambert*

Sandra Sagear certainly knew what it meant to struggle and overcome obstacles; but Sandy's family and friends remember her attitude, not her struggles. Sandy said, *"Can't* never did anything. *Can* did it all." She believed it and she lived it.

Sandy was born on March 22, 1950. She contracted polio at the age of seventeen months. Polio created limitations for her body, but Sandy's spirit and character created a hopeful and courageous life. It's hard to imagine the strength and tenacity required of a young girl who faced so many operations and extended hospital stays. It's not hard to imagine that Sandy must have felt frustrated or lonely at times; but she chose not to let people see that. She didn't ask for help when others thought she should; instead she chose to help others. She chose to push ahead, even when others wanted her to rest.

At the age of four, she was a March of Dimes Poster Girl. At 16, she was spokesperson for Plymouth Community Fund, (now known as United Way). She loved music. Like most teenagers, she loved the Beatles. While most teenagers watched the Beatles on Ed Sullivan, Sandy was backstage at Olympia Stadium watching the Beatles -- in a full body cast, no less.

Sandy's early education was completed at home with special tutoring. In 1965, she was able to attend East Middle School in Plymouth. In 1966, she went on to attend Plymouth High School, Central Middle School, (now, PARC). Once again, she displayed a creative tenacity in how she navigated a building without an elevator and a bus without a lift, wearing braces, using crutches, and carrying all her belongings.

Sandy graduated in 1969. After graduation, she worked as an office manager and became a computer whiz. She was known as an excellent student, valued employee, and a great friend.

More importantly, she was a loving and much-loved daughter, sister, and aunt. Sandy passed away on April 2, 1992, due to complications of pneumonia. She was 42 years old.

The Sandra Sagear Memorial Wall commemorates the perseverance and courage Sandy demonstrated throughout her life. It is dedicated to all of the students in our community that have shown the same kind of strength when faced with adversity."

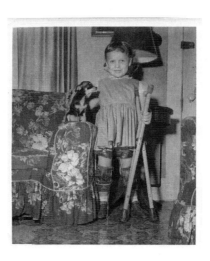

(Sandy Sagear. Permission to use granted by Vonnie Bench)

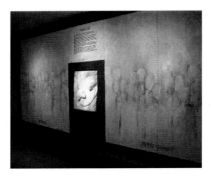

(Sandra Sagear Wall of Courage, designed and constructed by Dennis Jones.
Permission to use granted by Vonnie Bench and Dennis Jones)

(Sandra Sagear Wall of Courage, Plymouth High School, Canton Mi. Family: Tim & Donna Sagear, Vonnie & Jimmy Bench, Josh, Lisa, Violet Bench, Tiffany and James Lambert. Dennis Jones, Architect and Designer of the Sandra Sagear Wall of Courage, Co-chairs: Jerry Trumpka & Debra Madonna, The Sandra Sagear Wall of Courage, five Honorees. Rotary Club of Plymouth A.M. Sandra Sagear Scholarships, sixty-three Sagear Scholarships.)

Jerry Trumpka contracted polio when he was eight months old. Jerry was an essential part of the committee to build the Sandra Sagear Wall of Courage. Jerry felt a kinship with Sandy, even though he never met her, even though they had both been at the same Beatles concert. He wanted to see the day that polio was eradicated from the globe. Jerry was a doer of good deeds, more than anyone knew. On any given day, he was helping someone somewhere. He would have loved the Miracle League of Plymouth; he would have been one of the announcers. He was my pal and mentor. Jerry passed away from post-Polio Syndrome on March 17, 2008.

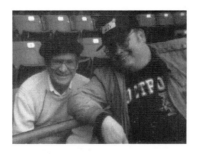

(Ernie Harwell & Jerry Trumpka.)

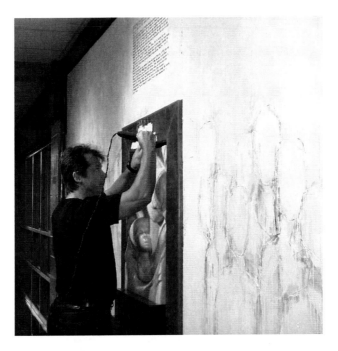

(*Dennis Jones, Sandra Sagear Wall of Courage. Plymouth High School, Canton, MI. Permission to use granted by Becky Trumpka and Dennis Jones*)

Frail as Butterfly Wings

SOME have a very strong opinion of what we should do when we have an illness. We want to be strong and dignified, but sometimes, the body is just worn out.

No one doubted that my grandfather, Bill, had a lot of spunk. He died at 98. Until the last two weeks of his life, he got dressed and went to the cafeteria for meals. A few nights before he died, he was eating applesauce. He told me it was the best applesauce that he ever had. I asked him I could have some. His answer, "No, get your own." He was playful and cantankerous. It was his nature from his beginning to his end.

My grandmother, Blanche, was so different. I would not use athletic, powerful and energetic to describe her. My grandmother was delicate, tender, and quiet. She was 4'11' and petite. Bill had a booming voice and he was not interrupted very often. Blanche crocheted doilies and afghans quietly. If she made a mistake, she ripped out what she had done. She grumbled and scowled until she retraced her steps to the point that she realized she had made a mistake. Then she was quiet again. She was a great cook and baker. She was famous for a chocolate cake with a seven-minute whipped frosting. I often stopped to see her in the afternoons and we watched soap operas; we talked, talked, talked and laughed.

The last few years of her life, she was frail and in constant pain. She was not the person who went outside and walked off the pain. She remained in a spot on the couch. I saw the pain on her face. When I visited, she always held my hand until I left. She held my hand not because she was in pain; my grandmother held my hand from the day I was born; she protected me. When she took my hand during the last days, she was just as tender.

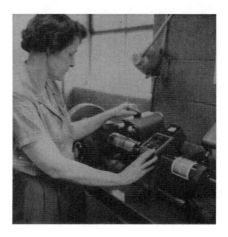

(Blanche working at the Plymouth Mail)

Jeff Good, When It Is Not You

RECOVERING from my stroke had challenges, but it was easier than watching someone you love go through pain and suffering. And it was easier than watching my brother go through things that little boys should never have to face. I am my brother's older sister, but about 15 years ago, I decided I would stop getting older and declared that he was the older brother.

While my 3-year-old brother was in another room with a chiropractor, the doctor stretched, pulled, and yanked his legs. I sat in the waiting room. I did not understand the pain he was experiencing, but I heard his pain. He was being tortured. When he was 5 or 6, my brother went into the hospital, stayed for weeks, several times. When he was in an operating room; his tendons were being cut and sliced. I did not hear anything because I could not be in the hospital or visit him. He came home covered with bandages and wearing bulky casts or hard braces. He returned to the hospital for more surgeries. His scars remained a reminder, in case he forgot. The pulling, yanking, cutting, and bracing did not accomplish a thing.

When he returned to the school's playground, he made it to the top of the slide wearing braces. Heaven help the kid who did not get down the slide as fast as possible because my brother was going down the slide, feet, and braces first. I wish I had a video of him, climbing the stairs to the top, maneuvering his body to get in a seated position, and then pushing off. I cringe thinking of Jeff's recently cut tendons, minimally protected by metal braces and shoes, colliding with the ground. I remember Jeff's best friend was cheering him on.

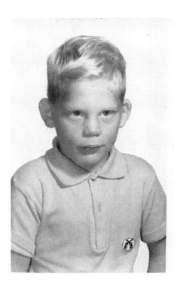

(My little brother, Jeff Good. Permission to use granted by Jeff Good)

Thoughts

Try Harder

If a child does not complete a task in a timely manner,
do you tell her, "Try Harder"?
If a child does not even start an assignment,
do you tell her, "Try Harder"?
This doesn't sound right. What are you trying to say?

If a child turns in a project with mistakes,
do you huff and puff and tell her,
"This is terrible. Try Harder"?
After you tell a little girl "Try Harder",
did you look her in the eyes?
Did your words help the little girl one little bit?

If the person packing your groceries is going too slow,
Do you tell her, "I am in a hurry"?
If you see a person struggle,
do you think out loud,
"What is the matter with her"?

If someone is recovering from this or that,
do you think it would help if you stood on a table
and yelled so the whole world hear your irritation,
"Heal Faster"?
This doesn't sound right. What are you trying to say?

A therapist does not look at her watch and say,
"Your appointment is 55 minutes, you only have 27 minutes left.
SPEED IT UP".
This doesn't sound right. What are you trying to say?

Do you tell the grass it is growing too fast?
Do you?

Do you tell your plants to grow larger flowers?
Have you thought to be patient and watch flowers bloom?
Have you?
No one at a library ever said, "Read Faster".
The people at my favorite stores, always greet me,
"I am happy to see you".

Let us trade in all our "Try Harders".
Look into someone's eyes and smile.
How long do you think it will take to get a smile back?
Demonstrate what "HURRY UP" looks like.
Demonstrate what "Take your Time" looks like.
Demonstrate what "I am here" looks like.

Give your time to others.
You have time because someone else gave you their time.
Remember that Any One who is living is brave.
Remember that Every One may have difficulty
putting one foot in front of the other.
I know you are doing the best that you can.
Aren't we all?
Me, too.
That is what I am saying.

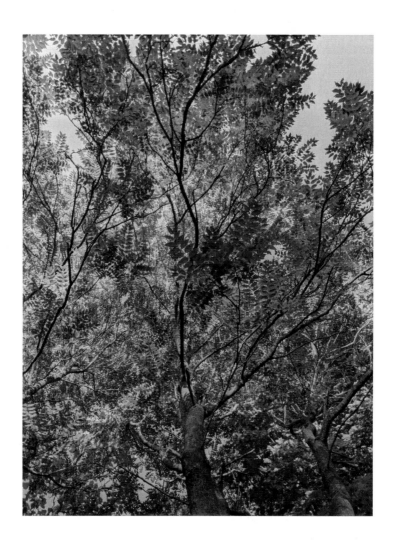

CHAPTER 11

The Power of Work and Play and We

January 2020

For Me

I worked on January 26, 2015. My business, QuixWorks Therapeutic Massage and Reiki, closed on January 27, 2015. In a world that is not perfect, imperfect humans should fit right in. Fact: I will die someday. On behalf of my ego, I wanted my family to know that I did a few things in my life. I do not want it to be said that I had a stroke and then I died. Geez, I want it known that between "stroke" and "dying", I walked, talked, did things I loved to do, and lived a good life. My plan or hope is that I earn this space every day that I am here in this world. I hope my husband, sons, daughters, and grandson confirm that while there was difficulty, there were happy times, too. I hope my family knows that having them by my side made everything possibly.

A Reckoning

I am grateful for all that was done for me. The care I received helped me succeed. I believed that I should do the same for others. I kept a journal, starting at six months post-stroke while everything was fresh in my mind. I included what happened to me since January 27, 2015, the day of my stroke. The recovery, plans for the future, as well as how I handled serious matters in the past—everything is there. No crying over what "I used to do," or "I used to be." A tear or two is acceptable; being a little sad is okay, too. I have stepped down from working for pay for medical reasons. My marketable skills are wobbly. I do not have a pension, just a social security allowance.

What do I do with my "What I Still Want to Do" list? What do I do with all this wisdom rattling around in my brain? I evaluated what I have done, who I have met along the way, what I have learned, and what is next. I have led an eclectic life and I want to continue. It suits my nature. Jobs, volunteering, finding money for good causes, and raising three sons brought me to today. There are people I have met that have changed me for the better; others have crawled into my heart and stayed forever.

Michigan
Plymouth State Home, (PSH), 1972 - 1973

PLYMOUTH State Home, aka Plymouth Center for Human Development, was a long-term care facility for "developmentally disabled and physically challenged" children and adults.

Before there were cars, it would take a day's ride on horseback to get from Detroit to 5 Mile Road and Sheldon, Plymouth and Northville. Even with a car, the drive from Detroit to Plymouth and Northville seemed like a long ride to the country. Many institutions were built a long ride from Detroit: Maybury Sanatorium, Wayne Country Training School, Hawthorne Center, Detroit House of Corrections (DeHoCo), Robert Scott Correction Facility, Northville Regional Psychiatric Hospital (Northville State Hospital) and Plymouth Center for Human Development (Plymouth State Home and Training School). Distance was one of the ways to deal with people who were didn't have a place in their homes and neighborhoods. Miles are not the only way to keep a distance from others.

Before you read this, this is not meant to reflect poorly on parents or families of the young people who lived at Plymouth State Home. The children placed at Plymouth State Home may not have been many miles from their home, their families, and schools their sisters and brothers attended. During the 1960s and 70s, families of children with "disabilities and handicaps" were often counseled to move a child from their home and community into a facility or institution. The "home away from" was not home. It was only "away from home."

They may have been advised not to visit because it would be hard for their child. The experts at the time pointed out that it would be burdensome to care for their child at home; it would be tough on the brothers and sisters. It may be difficult to get a doctor or dentist, or go church, and certainly, there was no place for them in schools. Parents may be told, "It is better this way," but it was not better. It was not better for the parents to be without their child or the child to be without their parents. Families had limited options. Parents never forgot their child. The longer that a child was separated from her parents, the child would have limited or no memory of their parent or what a parent was at all. Some parents chose to keep their children with them at home.

The people who built Plymouth State Hospital demonstrated that children and adults were institutionalized without an exit plan. Nothing changed until families fought to regain their rights as parents and their children's rights in the mid-1970s. Families fought to remind the world that the patients and residents who lived in these institutions were someone's child, brother, sister, grandchild, niece, nephew, cousin, or next door neighbor.

The complex opened in 1960 and closed in 1984. All the buildings have been torn down, replaced by houses, condos, senior citizen apartments, a strip mall, and a golf course. There is always money for what we want, but stingy when the money takes care of someone else. There is no mention of the children and adults who once lived there, no plaques, no wall of names.

I am not happy that these institutions existed. I worked in one. A book can never adequately describe the inside of these institutions. I am glad that I had the opportunity to spend time with the young people who lived there, I will never forget them. I always wished I had met their families. During my time at the hospital, the people I worked with were caring people, but we knew we could not replace the young people's families.

Orientation

I was assigned to a room with 7 or 8 children, served lunch, brushed teeth, bathed, and changed the children's clothes. One of the little boys was seated in a wooden chair, slanted back and no rollers. He was a beautiful little boy, 6 or 7 years old. This was the little boy's first day at the hospital; it was my first day working on the hospital unit.

A nurse and a woman came into the room while I was working. The nurse introduced me to the woman. She was the mother of the beautiful little boy seated in the wooden chair. The mother was weeping; the kind of crying that hurts your heart to hear. The mother hugged her little boy while he was still in the wooden chair. A few minutes later the nurse and the mother left the room, leaving her son, the other children, and myself.

During the afternoon's orientation session, I wanted to ask, "How many children are visited by their parents and how often?" I did not ask the question, but I learned that the answer was, "not often". They were not forbidden to visit, but the prevailing attitude was the children were better in an institution. It was painful for the families to visit their child in an institution; support for parents and alternatives were limited.

The mother of the little boy sitting in the wooden chair was crying; not the tears when you dropped your child off at school for 6 hours. This mother was crying the tears as she left her son in "this place" and she did not have a plan to return. The tears are different.

Howe 3

I was permanently assigned to Howe 3, a unit of 51 young people, 7 to 10 people per room. The residents / patients were 18 years and older, born in 1953 and older. Only two of the young people were mobile, four or five were verbal. They were placed onto a bed and that is where they lived. I was born in 1951. I was their peer. From my first day on the unit, they were children to me, who never had a childhood.

In my time on Howe 3, therapy was not provided for the children, not even simple range of motion exercises. I suspect no one thought that the children would live as long as they had. Nothing was done for them, excepting feeding, bathing and changing diapers, and clothes.

Paul and Richard

PAUL and Richard were precious little boys; they had been roommates for many years. They lived in cribs with very high sides, shiny silver bars, on wheels. Paul smiled from the time he woke up till he fell asleep. I suspect he smiled in his sleep, too. When he thought he had my attention, his smile was sweeter. Richard was grumpy. I discovered if I was silly and made Paul laugh, then Richard was less grumpy. Paul and Richard were unable to turn their heads. They lay on their backs and never on their tummies. It didn't take long to figure out how to change Paul's diapers and not block Richard's view of Paul. I learned the hard way that if I placed myself between them so Richard could not see Paul, he became upset. He made the sound of a lost little lamb looking for his mother. He could not be consoled until I moved Paul so Richard could see Paul again. Changing Richard's diapers created a problem. If I tipped Richard, he faced the wall and he could not see Paul. But if I tipped Richard, pushed and spun the crib around so that Paul was once again in view, then all was right in the world. It was a good thing I was in shape. I pushed the two cribs close to each other, but I learned later that pulling the cribs away from each other was distressing to the boys. I never knew why they had to pull the cribs away from each other. I would have left the cribs next to each other.

Why were the cribs pulled apart? Why not leave the cribs close together. There was no good reason except every crib had one side pushed up against a wall. Or the cribs had always been placed across from each other, not next to each other. Or it violated the fire code. Or there was no reason, good or otherwise.

Arts, Culture and Therapy

DURING my time at Howe 3, the young people received no art therapy, recreational therapy, occupational therapy, physical therapy, or simple, daily range of motion exercises. There were no volunteers, and only a few visitors. There were no announcements over a loud speaker. The voices they heard were of the few people who worked there.

There was music and baseball on the radio. In 1972–73, the available channels were 2, 4, 7, 9, maybe 50 and 56, spotty reception, no cable, just antennas. I read books and newspapers to the young people and told them stories. The television shows were *Rita Bell's Prize Movie, Bill Kennedy at the Movies and the Soaps.* My favorite was *All My Children.* Watergate Hearings took over the airwaves for months, alternating on three channels.

One morning, the movie on *Rita Bell's Prize Movie* was *Tale of Two Cities.* It gave me something to think about while I spent time in Howe 3. My home was just a few miles away.

"It was the best of times, it was the worst of times, it was the age of wisdom, it was the age of foolishness, it was the epoch of belief, it was the epoch of incredulity, it was the season of light, it was the season of darkness, it was the spring of hope, it was the winter of despair."

—Charles Dickens, *A Tale of Two Cities*

"It is a far, far better thing that I do, than I have ever done, it is a far, far better rest that I go to than I have ever known."

—Sydney Carton, Charles Dickens, *A Tale of Two Cities*

You may think having the television soap operas play in the young people's room was foolish, but for five days a week, we listened to Erika Kane's adventures and heard the drama of the Martin family. The voices were familiar and part of the day, five days a week. The Martins visited Howe 3 more than family visitors.

New Places, New Faces

PAUL and Richard were scheduled to leave Howe 3 soon after I left the job at Plymouth State Hospital, but they were not going home. Paul and Richard were being moved to different facilities, new "homes away from home."

When I walked out of the building on my last day, I knew I would never forget the young people I met. What I learned from them was the cornerstone of the path I took professionally and personally. This place, these faces pointed me back to college. I became an Occupational Therapist, Massage Therapist, Childbirth Education Instructor, Love and Logic Parenting Instructor, and a mother. If I ever had the opportunity to change anything, I wish I would have stayed longer. This was my beginning.

I learned to talk to young people who cannot speak. I was a guest in their world so I learned to speak their language: gentleness. If I brushed their teeth and combed their hair with gentleness, they spoke back with their eyes. If I told them a ridiculously hilarious story, they laughed with their eyes. If I was too busy doing something else, their eyes worked hard to let me know that I had ignored them. When I spoke to them, they spoke to be with their sweetness. Paul, Richard, the 49 other young people of Howe 3, and the little boy in the wooden chair will be with me forever. I put them in my pockets and carry them everywhere.

Northville State Psychiatric Hospital, Northville Center Adult Psychiatric Hospital (NSH)

YOU can learn everything about psychiatric patients from books, but is not like being in a psychiatric hospital. Northville State Psychiatric Hospital had a large population when I worked there in the mid-70s. But in the 1990s, Northville and other state psychiatric hospitals were emptied and shuttered. It was not that I wanted to see people in an institution, but after closing the hospitals, many patients were left with nowhere to go and inadequate support.

Northville State Hospital was not an ideal facility, but there must be alternatives and solutions other than leaving mentally ill people to fend for themselves.

Even if you do not understand mental health issues, we cannot turn our backs on human beings who struggle. Who decided to close the facilities and throw away the safety nets? It does not matter who is responsible, no one stopped it. The abandoned buildings still stand.

We All Deserve the Best Care

I have had the time to think of the care I received when I had the stroke and my recovery. I often thought of the people I cared for at Plymouth State Home and the folks at Northville State Hospital. Individuals were placed in a supervised setting to live; food and clothes were provided. If you stayed at a psychiatric hospital, the facility was predetermined by a patient's home address and a zip code; it wasn't predetermined by diagnosis. Even now a psychiatric patient will get services, but it is short-term and their families do not have the support they need.

If you have a car accident, a heart attack, or another emergency, someone calls 911 and an ambulance comes to wherever you are and you will be taken to the closest hospital. I, a 63-year-old woman, qualified for the best medical treatment available without asking. Part of my recovery included counseling, a plan and a list of people to provide me with whatever I needed. Without intervention, I would have struggled. Without long-term support, I would have been lost. Why is there the best help for physical issues? Why is there a fractured health system provided for those with mental health issues?

In the mid-70s, a mental health patient's admission and care was so different than a general medicine patient. Even now. What I know for sure is that if, upon arrival at the hospital January 2015, instead of treating me with care, treating my illness with urgency, I was placed on a bed, minimum medical treatment, no therapies, no plans, and my outcome would not have been the same. I know. I saw the results of benign neglect in children and adults at PSH and NSH.

Colorado

1983: We became parents. We moved to Colorado.

During my 20s, I spent time with people who were hidden in the shadows of health care. Living in Colorado, I would see a whole different view. The theme for the next eight years would be "Healthy Babies, Healthy Children, Healthy Parents, Healthy World, Prevention, Care" Version 1.0. I was happy.

Breathe

I began teaching prepared childbirth classes just before my third son was born. The classes took place in the hospital my second son was born in. My husband is a computer guy. Our sons are well-rounded, but they are proficient with technology. I am not sure what my sons thought of what I did for a living. Because I loved it, I would talk about it. My teaching props, charts, plastic pelvis, breast pumps and a blue knitted uterus often ended up on the kitchen table.

I had the opportunity to teach and support expectant parents about pregnancy, labor and babies. It is very important to be factual, but take into account the complexity of the emotions and physical changes they experience. I wanted to empower parents to care for and love themselves through it all. I reminded them to eat, drink water, sleep, exercise in their spare time, and go to regular doctor visits. One of the requirements of being a childbirth educator was to observe labors and delivery. It is not the same as having a baby myself, but it is pretty thrilling, very cool.

Pregnant Teenagers

WE lived in Jefferson County, Colorado. The county school district had a school-based program for school-aged young adults who became pregnant. They were moved to a central school equipped to allow these young women to remain in school before and after their baby is born. While the mom is in school, there is a day care on site for the babies. I taught classes at the school to discuss pregnancy, labor, and delivery. We talked about babies, how to care for themselves and their baby. We did not discuss whether or not they kept their child or were giving the baby up for adoption; that was a discussion they had with their family and counselors. I brought badly-needed factual information about pregnancy and babies into this classroom. I needed to balance the presentation of this material against the complex emotions and physical changes these young women experience. I wanted them to be empowered, to love themselves through it all, handled with care and kindness. It does not matter how old a woman is when she has a baby, it is a unique experience for everyone.

Club Crest Babysitting Coop

WE made so many dear friends in Colorado, thanks to the Club Crest Babysitting Coop. There were no other people that I wanted to hang with or leave my children with and vice versa. I knew all about babies, but I did not really know about staying home with little ones, all day, every day.

Just before my second son was born, my prenatal exercise instructor, Nancy Smith, asked me if I would like to trade time babysitting for each other. Next, Nancy and I would ask women in grocery stores or the park if they would like to trade time and babysitting each other's children. Everyone who said yes asked other mothers they knew. That was it. We ended up with about twenty to twenty five families with one child, two, or three children.

It was not a cult. It was an awakening and a friendship that only mothers have. This movement was about learning to take care of children and their mothers and fathers. Some mothers knew everything about teething, toilet training, and sharing; others knew a lot about other things. If you were sick, someone would deliver food and leave it on your doorstep. We carpooled. Even if we did not have an appointment, we could get a few hours to ourselves. This all took place before the internet and phones that send messages. We had phones with a cord to the wall.

My friends threw me a baby shower for Mark, son #3. Marcy Lamberson gave me a great big box of prepared food, individual servings which could be microwaved. She gift-wrapped the box. I kept that wrapped box in my freezer for a long time, a reminder of a friend and helpers. This extraordinary group of women could circle the wagons when times were tough, scary, when you were exhausted, wrestling with all the normal kids stuff and pregnancy adventures. And yes, even mothers in a babysitting coop could have a miscarriage. You would be treated with compassion and your kids were in good hands for as long as you needed.

This group was fun. Other mothers and fathers, laughing, crying, and becoming lifelong friends. I have kept in touch with several of the families, moms and kids. It has been a treat to watch the little kids I knew grow up and have adventures; some have children who look exactly like them.

(Marcy Lamberson. Melody Roe, Nancy Smith, Marcia Charles, Kathy Bird, Helen Maloney, Marya Biesendorfer. Cindy Calka Duba, Martha Jones, Shelley Christianson, Cindy Churchill, Susan Schubert, Kim Giarratano, husbands and children.)

We

WHEN your little one becomes ill for a long time, long enough to worry parents, long enough for friends to check in on you, the concern and worry you feel stays with you for a lifetime. Friends know that mothers and fathers understand when something is wrong. Children know too. Friends know when you are up at 2 a.m., sitting on the stairs, reading books, looking for answers. Friends would let you feel terrible till you did not feel terrible anymore. Friends understand frantic. Friends did not stop you from feeling frantic; they helped you do whatever you had to do for your child. Friends may not stop the worry, but you can trust them. Friends made it safe to go find answers and the kind of help that helps.

One day, my friend, Kim Giarratano, asked me what the doctor said about my little boy, Mark. I said, "She said, 'We'll check him at his 2-year checkup.'" Kim picked up my little boy and stood him on the kitchen island. "He won't last that long. *We* will get him well." *We* did get him well. She showered me the power of "*we*".

I told my husband that I was going to the library. I would be home when I found what I needed. Sitting on the floor, I pulled books off the shelf, looked through the index, read more, closed the book, grabbed another book. A lady stood next to me. She had beautiful red hair. She asked me questions. We talked for a long time. She took books from the shelf and gave them to me. She wrote in a notebook and handed me a piece of paper with the name of a doctor and books that she recommended. She asked me, "What is your little boy's name?" She said, "You will get Mark well." I wanted to thank her, but I could not find her. I told my husband what happened. I said, "She's a library angel. I needed this." He said, "You deserved this."

Adults are not the only ones you can lean on. We had put our Christmas tree up, but days went by and the tree was still bare. I was overwhelmed with worry. While I was at work, my older boys, Andrew and John decorated the tree. It was the prettiest tree ever. Seeing that tree, my worry melted away. I am not including the details of my son's condition because that is his story. Happily, he's well and has been for many years. My part of the story was to know how to cry, "Help." We were able to find reliable medical people who stayed with us till our son was better and who listened to us, the parents. I never worried that I would try crazy things; my posse helped me keep my worry in check.

We left our home in Colorado and moved back to Michigan. I missed all the moms who helped me be the best mom I could be. I miss them still. The lesson that I learned was to find a posse to be my side, wherever I live, while my children were growing up, and maybe when they are all grown up.

Michigan

WE moved back to Michigan. Simon and Garfunkel's "America" played on the radio. Our three sons grew and grew and grew older and taller. They went to school, graduated, went to college, graduated, and started their families. (Note: "their families" were also a part of our family.) My techie husband built our house. Quiz: How many computers does one person need? More than you might think.

"Healthy Babies, Healthy Mothers, Healthy Parents, Healthy Brothers and Sisters, Healthy Seniors, Healthy Every One, Healthy World", Version 2.0. I worked at St. Mary Mercy Hospital, Marion Women Center. I continued to talk to people about babies, their lives, happy times, stressful times, and worrisome times. In any given week, I taught a prepared childbirth class, parenting classes; take expectant parents on a tour of the maternity center, and a menopause group. It was quite an education for me. It was amazing how much I learned from others while I was teaching them. This is what I got to do on any given day or evening at St. Mary Mercy Hospital, Livonia, Michigan, thanks to of my co-workers in the Marian Women's Center Mary Jane Peck, Mary Lou Anolich, Teresa Doherty, Cheryl Grougan, Charlene Shedd, Nancy Mazur, and Carol Ann Fausone, Retired Brigadier General. Thank you.)

- taught Prepared Childbirth Classes
- observed Births
- taught Sibling Classes
- taught Infant Care Classes
- led Maternity Center Tours
- facilitated Love and Logic Parenting Classes
- taught Prenatal Exercise Classes
- facilitated Menopause Support Groups
- facilitated Breast Cancer Support Groups
- administered Bone Density Screening
- administered Blood Pressure Testing
- offered Chair Massages at Ladies Night Out

- worked as an Occupational Therapist, COTA, on the Behavioral Medicine Unit

What did I do at work today? I talked to expectant parents about having a baby, giggled about hot flashes, dealing with cancer, how to raise responsible children, or watched a baby being born. Being in the room when a baby comes is the best place to be. Everyone in the room is focused on the mother and the baby who is about to be born. A baby's head crowns, slowly emerging and, as magnificent that is, during the next seconds or minute, waiting for the baby to take his first breath, second breath, and then a cry. Well, in those few minutes, that baby courageously tells the world, "I am here." And the mother has let her baby go into the world. Not all births are perfect and mothers and babies can get into a rough spot. The one thing does not change; the helpers in the room are right there using all their knowledge to help mom and baby safe.

I have met a lot of pregnant moms and dads. I tell them the same thing. I do not know how they will do in school, if they will be a baseball player, or hate peas, but I know they will have a beautiful baby. They are not beautiful because they have lots of hair or no hair, skinny or plump. Look into a baby's eyes. That is where the beauty is.

What did you do at work today?

Menopause Support Group

I was privileged to host a Menopause Support Group at St. Mary's Hospital. This group met once a month. Guest speakers presented information on different medical issues, anything that women wanted information about: Hot Flashes, Hormone Replacement Therapy, Heart Health, Insomnia, and Incontinence were just some of the topics. And women could ask the doctors questions

Most people in this group did not like hot flashes. We reviewed all the latest information and discussed ways to deal with HF. Example: a woman and a man are sitting at a conference table. The woman begins to sweat, sweat rolling down her forehead, her neck. She does not say, "Is it hot in here or is it me?" because she is embarrassed. She discreetly mops her brow. She was fairly confident that it is a hot flash because she has them all the time. The man begins to sweat and he asks, "Is it hot in here or is it me?" Someone calls 911 because he may be having a heart attack. I liked hot flashes. I felt refreshed. It felt like my body was getting bad toxins out of my system. It was my own spa. **Important:** Get a regular check-up. Consult with your doctor. Never ignore symptoms a woman is having.

Some women report that they feel grumpy, crabby and cantankerous. Grumpiness serves a purpose. If you are really crabby, people may stay away from you; then you can focus on taking care of yourself. The 40s and 50s are the time in our lives that we can assess our health, both physical and emotional. We can make plans for the rest of our lives. As we age, we need to like ourselves or learn to like ourselves because we are going to be with ourselves for a long, long time.

A Missed Opportunity

LOOKING back, I missed an opportunity. When I worked at St. Mary Mercy Hospital, I should have suggested a class about "Brains", "Brain Health", or a "Brain Support Group". The group would be for people with a brain disorders, families, caregivers, or those who just want to know about the brain. There would be guest speakers. The class would cover:

- Normal Aging and the Brain

- Anatomy of the Brain

- Brain Disorders such Alzheimer's Disease, Dementias, Strokes and TIAs, Traumatic Brain Injury, Epilepsy, Seizure Disorders, Parkinson's Disease, other Movement Disorders, Brain Cancer, Migraines, and Autism.

- The similarities and differences between the healthy brain and brain disorders.

If you think that lay people wouldn't be able to understand, parents are lay people and know much more about having babies than doctors did 60 years ago. It would be helpful to those who are dealing with brain issues; not knowing, costs everyone. Not all brain disorders can be prevented and there are many unknowns. There are disorders that benefit by controlling blood pressure, protecting the brain by wearing helmets, and seatbelts. There is much more to learn and discover. It is helpful to know as much about the brain before there are issues. If you ask someone, what can you do to help slow Alzheimer's Disease or Memory Issues, the answer you may get is puzzles and crossword puzzles. There are more things that can be done to care for our brains.

Why did I not think of this before? After all, I had children and taught prepared childbirth classes; I had children and I taught parenting classes; I had a hot flash or two; I have a brain and had a stroke. I did not only depend on those experiences to teach a class; I learned everything I could and taught what I knew as of that day and always updated what I knew. I would have a model of a brain and charts. I had a plastic pelvis and a knitted uterus for the prepared childbirth classes. Maybe the class would be called **"NeuroPause"**. Gosh, I would have loved facilitating a Brain Class. When would be the next time be that I could talk about thalamus, basal ganglia and all the rest.

Summers, Music, and Baseball
Music in the Park (MiP) / Plymouth Community Arts Council (PCAC)

MUSIC in the Park began 1984. My time as the Chairwoman was 1994 – 2015. On summer Wednesdays at noon in Kellogg Park there are free-to-the-community concerts for children and their families, crowds of 1,000 to 3,000 people each week. For one hour a week, children, parents, grandparents with picnic lunches gathered in a park in the middle of town for singing, dancing, and making happy memories. I was the chairperson for 21 years. My sons helped me when they were younger. My job was to keep the rain away on concert days, make sure everyone was having a good time and reunite lost parents with their children. Occasionally, I announced when a parent wandered away from their child; no more music until the child found their lost parent.

Kellogg Park is in the middle of town, lots of trees, perfect for children, families, grandparents and music. When asked why he sponsored MiP, Carl Schultz said he just wanted to do something for the people who lived in Plymouth, and those that worked and visited Plymouth. Fact:

There are more strollers per capita on summer Wednesdays at noon in Kellogg Park than just about any other park.

(Thank you: Lisa Howard, Tyler Howard, Katie Howard, Nick Bair, Emily Bair, Christina and Derek Bair, Dick and Damaris "Dee" Schulte, Joanne Winkleman Hulce, Suzanne Parent, Flossie Ernzen, Tammy and Jeremy Trudelle, Sheila Paton, Patrick Olson, David Williamson, Ted Williamson, Charlie Stout, Jeff Burda, Bill Lawton, Mike Ager, The Wilcox Foundation: Win Schrader, Dan Herriman, Scott Dodge, Carl Schultz and family; City of Plymouth, Commissioners, Paul Sincock, City Manager, City of Plymouth Support Staff, Police, and Firemen.)

Some of MiP Musicians Over the Years

Guy Louis Sferlazza, Beverly Meyer, The Music Lady, Gemini, Las and San Slomovits and Emily Slomovits, Josh White Jr., Matt Watroba, Robert Jones, Saline Fiddlers, Barbara Hutchison, Jan Krist, Kitty Donohoe, Mustard's Retreat, Joel Tacey, Tom Seley, Gordon Russ, Jeremy Kittel, Cats and Fiddlers, Mike Ager and All Directions, Donna Novak, HarpBeat, Corwin Stout, elmoTHUMM, Paula Messner, Candy Band, Sarah Lenore, Zac Morgan, Phoenix, Joe Reilly, Plymouth – Canton Fife and Drum Core, Earth Angels. Marc Thomas & Max the Moose, and more.

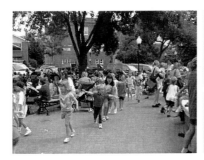 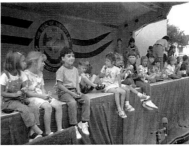

(A Summer Wednesday Music in the Park, (MiP 1999)

Thank Heaven for First Responders, Music and Sunshine

IT could not have been a prettier day on this sunny summer Wednesday, in Kellogg Park. The sun was bright. It was warm, but not too hot. The park was full of people who had come to Music in the Park, the Wednesday afternoon concert. Five months ago, I was not sure if I would be able to come back to this park. I did not want to be there if I was gloomy. I was overwhelmed. My friend, Jamie Jones, said that I would make it to the park. She was right. She is always right; it was a good day.

It was time to start the show. For 21 years, I organized these musical (and magical) concerts, ten times every summer. At the start of a concert, I welcomed everyone on behalf of the Plymouth Community Arts Council, thanked the sponsors and introduced the performer. This Wednesday was different, I welcomed everyone to Kellogg Park, but Jennifer and Lisa announced the sponsors. Guy

Louis Sferlazza had been part of the summer Wednesday concert lineup for a thousand years. Guy took my hand and I introduced him. Kellogg Park was full. I wanted to say how glad I was to be in the park. I do not think I said all that. It was very reassuring to feel better.

When I walked off stage, one of the firemen, Captain Jim Davison, told me that I looked better than I did the last time he saw me. He had been one of the rescue workers who helped me on the day of my health adventure and he made sure it was a safe trip to the hospital. Even today, he is the only person that makes me cry and I cry every time I see him. All the good emotions that had been keeping a low profile since January, jumped out like fireworks.

One year later, June 2016, I was no longer working on the Music in the Park program, but Marcel and I were in the park with our grandson, Teddy, in a stroller of course. It was our grandson's first MiP concert. I had waited a long time to take my grandbaby to a concert like my friends. To cap off my years in the park, I asked if I could go on stage and introduce the performer, Guy, and my beautiful grandson, Teddy, to the audience. That was a great way to step away from a place that had brought me so much happiness.

That was the day I knew I was going to be well and happy.

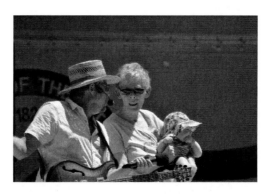

(Guy Louis Sferlazza, Deb, Teddy, Music in the Park, Kellogg Park.
Permission to use granted by Guy Louis Sferlazza,
Andrew and Justine Madonna)

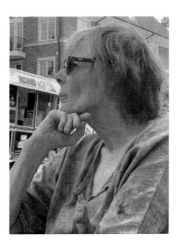

(at Music in the Park Aug. 11, 2021 with Jamie Jones and family.
I feel well and I am happy. I am home)

Miracle League Baseball of Plymouth (MLP)

MLP is played on the Bilkie Family Field, a baseball field, safe and accessible, for children and adults with special needs. "Every Child Deserves A Chance To Play Baseball" is the guiding principle. Before construction began, before the project had final approval, this baseball league was real to me. I dreamed about this field all the time, but children can't play real baseball in my dreams. There is nothing better for an adult to do to than to provide a place for children to play. The children may not know who built it, but they have a place to belong and play with others. The Bilkie Family Field is home to MLP and many children and adults that had never played baseball and never been part of a team.

On Opening Day, August 20, 2011, I was so excited. I walked a foot off the ground. My feet have not touched the ground yet. It was more spectacular than I imagined. MLP is the prettiest little baseball field anywhere. When I arrive at a game, I am happy. At the end of the day, I am even happier. Tom Hanks, in his memorable role as Coach Jimmy Dugan in *A League Of Their Own* said "There's no crying in baseball." He was absolutely right, but there are a lot of happy, overwhelming tears.

Have you ever been to a baseball game where everybody cheers every player, coach, buddies, umpires, announcers, and fans-in-stands? There is no booing in Miracle League baseball. No child is dropped off for a game; in fact, players bring their own cheering section. Volunteers often stay for two games, three games or four games.

The field was designed with features of a major league stadium from walking under the Bilkie Family Field sign, through the porch, into the sunlight, and lo and behold, there is the field.

- Everything to do with MLP is a joy. The only difficulty is finding a way to properly acknowledge and thank each and everyone for what they do to makes this baseball league real.

- Every Player has a Buddy to help him or her as little or as much as they need and to have fun.

- Coaches for each team

- Eight teams, four games a week, seven games in the spring, seven games in the fall

- Every player gets a set of baseball cards with their picture on it.

- An announcer who treats every game as if it is the bottom of the 9th inning in Game 7 of the World Series and each player is a champion.

- Umpires who keep the players safe and welcomes them home.

- Volunteers, Volunteers, Volunteers

- Sponsors

- Covered bleachers for all the fans

- A concession stand

- Spirit wear

- A picnic pavilion and picnic tables

- The sign on the Wishing Well is "All are welcome at this spot. Conjure up good wishes and thoughts, as many as you want or needed. When it comes time to leave, take wishes with you or leave one or two behind. Wishing tip: Wishes are powerful when shared with others."

- Egg Hunt, Trick or Treating on the Bilkie Family Field, walking in the 4th of July parade, and a Holiday Party.

- Bowling, Yoga, Dance.

- Mascots: every year we introduce mascots, stuffed animals, each with a name and a story. The first year, a mascot was named after Sandy Sagear's dog, Jingles. A bear named "Buddy" was named after Jerry Trumpka.

- An adult changing table was added a few years ago. Parents requested it. During the planning stage of the project, we had not thought of the needs of some of the older players. Thanks to the Shaw Construction, Ted Barker and Ted Mazaris; they found a way to retrofit the table in an existing restroom. I'm proud of that addition.

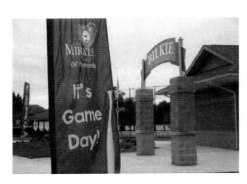 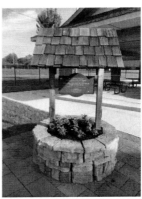

(Miracle League of Plymouth, the Bilkie Family Field, Plymouth MI)

MLP is a member of Miracle League, Conyers, Ga. MLP began under the umbrella of Rotary Club of Plymouth A.M., co-chairmen: Bob Bilkie and I. The groundbreaking took place on April 29, 2011, located on Theodore St., behind Central Middle School / the old Plymouth High School property. Funds to build MLP, support players, cover ongoing operations, and maintenance of the field come from good will, time, and generous donations from individuals, businesses, service organizations, and grants. When people heard about this baseball field, they asked, "What can I do to help?" And they did.

Upon completion of the field, Miracle League of Plymouth became an independent organization operated by co-founders Robert, Shari Bilkie, Amanda Lehnert, and family, Debra & Marcel Madonna, Mark Madonna. In addition, Kevin Finnerty, Geoff Taylor, John Gasloli, Stacey Diefenbach, Wendy Williamson, Kelly Herman, and Sam Plymale who watch over MLP.

- Steve Anderson, City of Plymouth Recreation.

- Shaw Construction, Manager, Ted Barker, Site Manager and, Ted Mazaris.

- Architect: Joseph Philips. Engineer: Mike Bailey.

- With affection and gratitude: every Player, every Family, every Friend, every Fan, every Grandma and Grandpa, every Volunteer, every Coach, every Umpire, every Announcer, every Photographer, every Supporter, and every Donor. Thanks to everyone who built the prettiest baseball field anywhere.

- Special guests: Michigan Paralyzed Veterans of America

- Marcel Madonna and Mark Madonna: Everything you did to make this dream come true.

- My dear friends, Bob and Lynne Hendzell

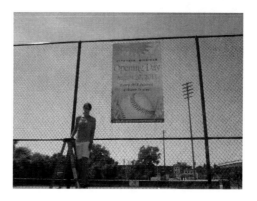

(Lisa Howard, artist, and Executive Director, Plymouth Community Arts Council, hanging the banner she made for MLP, Opening Day, August 20, 2011. Permission to use granted by Lisa Howard)

I'm a COTA, Certified Occupational Therapist Assistant. I received an Associate's Degree at Schoolcraft College, It's been very special to me to be part of this Miracle League. Some children and adults hadn't had the opportunity to play a sport and be a part of a team. If there were physical or emotional reasons that a children and adults hadn't been able to play on a traditional baseball field, Miracle League fields are accessible and safe for everyone. If the children and adults, need more help than she would have on a traditional baseball field, well there are buddies for everyone. We wanted parents and families to sit in the bleachers, watch and cheer their children and talk to other parents.

It tickles me because we have been able to tell people that this little baseball field was therapeutic for so many children and adults to play and play with others and everyone to watch. People listened. Maybe they hadn't thought of the importance of playing with others before; but once they have visited MLP, they understood; I have always thought that MLP was Occupational Therapy for the community. I hope a picture of the Miracle League of Plymouth baseball field, filled with players, family, and volunteers may someday be on the front cover of *O.T. Practice.*

Is play important for children? Yes, play is indispensable. And I know what happens if a child doesn't have the chance to move around and play, and play with others. I know. I have seen it. At the first game of the fall season this year, (August 14, 2021), the tenth anniversary of MLP, my son, John, observed that most of MLP's younger players were born into a world that has always had Miracle League baseball. Yes, there is crying in baseball.

"Every Child Deserves A Chance To Play Baseball"

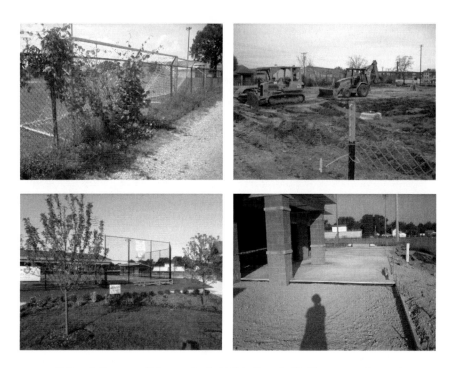

(Miracle League of Plymouth, the Bilkie Family Field, 2010 and 2011)

Telling Stories
Michigan
Plymouth Canton Observer, bi-weekly column, Around Town, 2004-2005

I have been involved in different activities in the community: a parent volunteer in the schools and the Plymouth Community Arts Council's Music in the Park.

I would be one of the people who got the word out an event. I sent out press releases to the media, including *The Plymouth and Canton Observers*. There was a time when the local newspapers were the best way to publicize activities. The Observer coverage of groups and events was critical to the success of activities. They did not just tell you when an event was taking place, but they told the story behind the event.

Brad Kadrich and Joanne Maliszewski, editors of the *Plymouth and Canton Observer*, invited me to a meeting at Panera Bread. They asked me if I would be interested in writing a column, about whatever I wanted. Holy cow, yes I was very interested. It was a dream comes true. The column, *Around Town*, 750 words, was on the front page of the second section, down the entire left side. For the next 18 months, my column appeared bi-weekly in the *Observer*. P.S. Important. I was paid to write a column for a newspaper. Ta Da.

My grandparents, Bill and Blanche, worked at the Plymouth Mail, which later became the Plymouth Observer. Bill's job was to make sure the newspaper presses worked. Before automation, Blanche inserted advertisements into each newspaper. When I was two and three years old, Blanche took me to work with her. I sat on a table with pencil and paper, happy to spend time with my grandma and her co-workers. I do not know if the Plymouth Mail knew they offered day-care. That was what I wrote about in the column, nice people who workedwith and for others to make their town a good place to live.

Michigan
WSDP, Wednesdays at 10:30 a.m. 2008 – 2013

WSDP 88.1 FM, Plymouth-Canton Schools, a student run radio station, is a jewel. Tune in and hear for yourself. My son, Mark, was on the staff of WSDP for all 4 high school years, hosting his own show every Tuesday afternoon. It was a treat to be driving around and hear my son on the radio.

There was one radio show, hosted by a non-teenager named Betty Smith about things in the community, in particular, senior citizens. I loved her show.

Betty was fascinating, like all the people and things she likes, especially jazz. Her guests on the show reflected that. Betty hosted the show for 10 years. I received a call from Betty one day. She was stepping down from the show because she had things she wanted to do, including writing a book. She wrote that book, *Beti's Book*.

Betty Smith and Bill Keith, WSDP Station Manager, asked me if I would like to step into Betty's time slot. I was fifty seven, not quite a senior citizen and not a teenager or a high school senior. I followed a similar format as Betty Smith's show *Lemonade with BJ*, but expanded it to all ages.

2008 - 2013, I hosted a show, inviting people from the Plymouth-Canton area to be a guest on the show and talk about the things they did to make the community a good place to live. The show was a half hour on Wednesdays at 10:30 a.m. I called it *Community*. The show started with my theme song, "Here Comes the Sun" because it is always my theme song. At the fifteen-minute break and the end of the show, I chose the music that played. Bill taped the shows so that the guests would have a copy and one for my family. Because people are often busy on Wednesdays at 10:30, Marcel posted the radio shows on line.

P.S. I was not paid, but I played music and talked to people on the radio. It was cool.

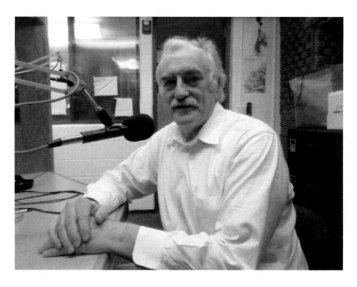

(Marcel, my Last Guest on my Last Show, WSDP)

Michigan
Helpers, Friendraisers, Awareness Raisers, Fundraisers, Preservers, Recyclers, Carpoolers, Volunteers, and Caregivers

IT starts with picking up a piece of paper on ground and placing in the proper receptacle, without being asked. You give a friend's child a ride to baseball practice when you are asked. Your friend says, "Thanks. I was in a bind. You really helped me." You say, "I was glad to do it". Parents are needed to go with your child's class to Greenfield Village." Once you sign your name to one Field Trip Parents sheet, you are a sure thing for all the extras at school.

Most people I know give and help wherever needed. In our town, children and teens pitch in. Volunteers are valuable, whether they help at school, in the neighborhood, or in our town. It takes more than money to make a town a good place to live. That is where the residents, business, and service organizations come together. PTA parents are dynamite; they raise money, clean up playgrounds, and provide money to teachers to spend on classroom supplies because PTA parents know teachers spend their own money for their students and classrooms.

My son's first grade teacher had set out the Sign-Up Sheets at her classroom Open House. I evaluated what I could do and then I saw it. I stopped. Taking the pencil, I happily signed my name on the "Reading Mom" Sign Up sheet. I was going to be back in first grade, helping children with their reading. When I was in first grade, my teacher, Miss Smart, asked children who could read to help those who struggled. I was back in first grade and reading. Ta Da.

Sometimes, the need is money and more money. There seems never to be enough money for health-related research and treatment costs. There are fundraisers for all types of causes and the need is the same: money, money and raise awareness. We walk, walk, walk, run, ride bikes, wear red, wear purple, shave our heads, or let our hair grow and donate our locks.

If the cause is personal, we have to do something to address our sadness, anger, and grief. We have to do something because doing nothing is too painful and heartbreaking so we stand, sit, ride, and walk with others. Things I did once upon a time.

Occupational Therapist, Schoolcraft College, Massage Therapist, Schoolcraft College, Reiki Master, Prepared Childbirth Educator, Plymouth State Home, Plymouth Center for Human Development for children and adults, Northville State Hospital, an adult psychiatric hospital, Club Crest Babysitting Coop, Prepared Childbirth Classes, Lutheran Medical Center, Jefferson County Schools, a school based program, childbirth education for pregnant teenagers, Livonia Childbirth Education Association.

St. Mary Mercy Hospital, Marion Women Center: Prepared Childbirth Classes, Observe Births, Sibling Classes, Infant Care Classes, Maternity Center Tours, Prenatal Exercise Classes, Parenting Classes, Menopause Support Groups, Menopause Support Groups, Breast Cancer Support Group, Bone Density Screening, Blood Pressure Testing, Behavioral Medicine Unit.

QuixWorks Therapeutic Massage and Reiki. (Tricia Kennedy, Sherry Lorimer, Lauren Gohl, Donna Farr, Erin Quillman, Michelle Clemens. Located next to Dairy King), Futures Health Core – Occupational Therapy, Plymouth Community Arts Council, Board Officer and President, Art Mom, Music in the Park (MiP), Plymouth Community Arts Council, (PCAC), Chairperson, Miracle League of Plymouth Baseball, (MLP), President, Commissioner , Damaris Fine Arts Award, Plymouth Community Arts Council, (PCAC).

Sandra Sagear Wall of Courage, Plymouth High School, Canton Mi. Plymouth-Canton Observer, Bi-Weekly Column, *Around Town*. WSDP, 8.1, High School radio station, weekly show, *Community*. PARC Committee, Plymouth Arts & Recreation, "Saving Central Middle School". The Susan G. Komen 3-Day Breast Cancer Walk, Team "Hearts for Gretchen". St. Baldrick's Foundation. ALS Ice Bucket Challenge, Karmanos Cancer Institute, H.O.T. (Hazards of Tobacco), West Board & Volunteer, Legendary Locals of Michigan by Leis Dauzet-Miller, Ruth Whipple Huston Award, City of Plymouth, Inaugural Notable PHS Graduate, Parent Involvement Committee, PCEP.

Parent Volunteer, Allen School, Field Trip Mom, Reading Mom, etc. , Parent Volunteer, Central Middle School, Parent Involvement Committee, PCEP.

**St. Baldrick's Foundation fundraiser to fight childhood cancers
was held at the Plymouth Roc, May 18, 2014.**

(Permission to use granted by Rachel Koelzer, Andrew Madonna,
Mark Madonna, Eric Bacyinski, Angela Nolan)

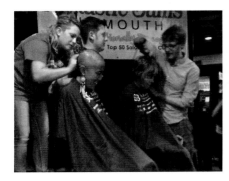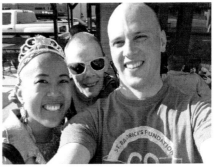

*(Rachel Koelzer, Andrew, Deb, Mark, Rachel Koelzer, Deb, Eric Bacyinski.
Michael Siegrist and Alice McCardell not picture)*

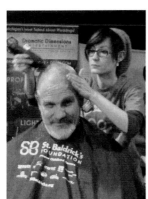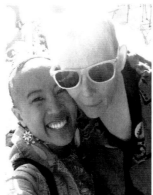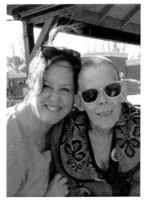

(Brad Kadrich, Rachel, Deb, Angela Nolan and Deb. Thank you)

ALS Ice Bucket Challenge raises awareness and funds for research Amotrophic Lateral Sclerosis. The event took place after Music in the Park, Kellogg Park, August 20, 2014.

(Permission to use granted by Abigail Samuels, Rob Parent, Eric Bacyinski, Lisa Howard, Guy Louis Sferlazza, Colleen Abb)

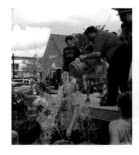
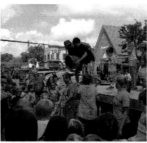
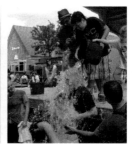

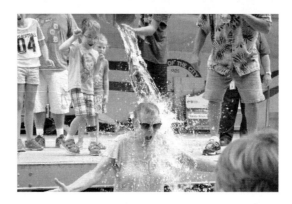

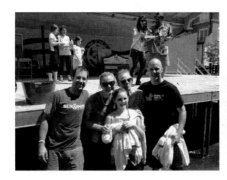
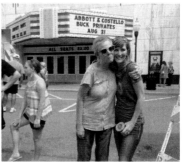

(Abigail Samuels, in blue,Rob Parent, Eric and Brooke Bacyinski, Deb,Water Pourers, Mason and Gavin, Helpers, Alexa and Skylar, (Front: Rob Parent, Abigail Samuels, Brooke Bacyinski, Deb, Eric Bacyinski. Back: Lisa Howard, Guy Louis Sferlazza. And Deb and Colleen Abb. Thank you,)

Hearts for Gretchen

(The Susan G. Komen 3-Day Breast Cancer Walk
raises funds and awareness to fight breast cancer, September 2008.
Team "Hearts for Gretchen" in honor of Gretchen Little)

(Permission to use granted by Jack Pitluk)

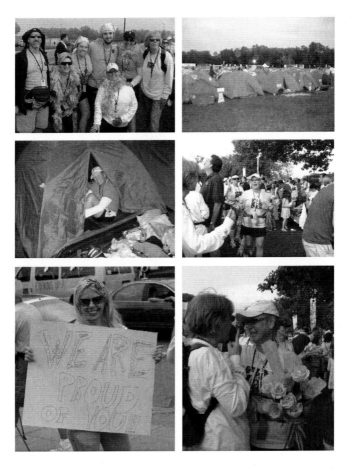

*(Hearts for Gretchen Team, Suzie Pitluk, (Gretchen Little's sister),
Gretchen Pitluk (Suzie's daughter), Nathan Pitluk (Suzie's son),
Eric Surprenant, Elena Surprenant, Linda Brunetto, and Jack Pitluk,
our team's wingman. Tricia Kennedy, Cheerleader. Suzie Pitluk, Deb,
"The Finish". Suzie Pitluk, Deb, "We did it".)*

Thoughts

I Wanted to Be Everything

I have been *"Everything,"*
but it was not a good idea at all.
I always wanted to be a doctor,
a pediatrician, a neurologist. a neurobiologist,
a kinesiologist, and an occupational therapist.
I mean I wanted to be a doctor so much
that I sometimes think that I am a doctor,
with no license, with no degree,
but a doctor nonetheless.

doctors, nurses, and all the rest must be smart,
confident, competent, caring,
extremely, supremely competent,
kind,
and, for heaven's sakes, please,
be curious.
be so curious that you never say, "I don't know"
without a "yet" at the end of a sentence
or "I don't know, but I am going to think about this."

the experience of being a patient has reminded me
of the necessity of changing my specialty to a Doctor of Demystification.
a Demystifier elucidates, illuminates, simplifies, interprets, illustrates.
a Demystifier explains the scary stuff.
an empathetic Demystifier clarifies everything
in a language you can understand.

a Demystifier does not always use words.

a Demystifier may hold your hand.

a Demystifier gives you time with facts.

a Demystifier gives you time and quiet.

a Demystifier sits by your side for as long as needed.

a Demystifier may not be a doctor, but it helps if a doctor is a Demystifier.

a doctor of Curiosity and Demystification. Yes, that's me.

or maybe I could be a Crossing Guard and a Fairy Godmother

and make the world a safe and healthy place for children,

a place where children can blossom, grow strong,

be healthy, loved,

and play, play, play,

until it's time to go to bed and have sweet dreams.

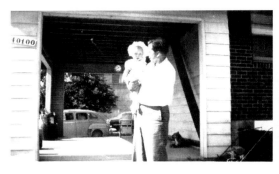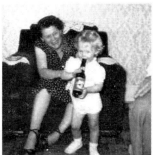

(Bill and Deb. Blanche and Deb.)

Peace

CHAPTER 12

THE POWER OF ACKNOWLEDGMENTS, APPRECIATION, AND GRATITUDE

ON January 27, 2015, I started my day, like most days in an upright position, driving somewhere. Mid-morning that changed. I could breathe without assistance, but I could do nothing voluntarily. As I woke up, I listened to the person who was nearest. If no one was telling me what to do, I rested. I wasn't afraid or distracted. I didn't have anything else to do. There was nothing on my calendar that was more important than what I was doing. For the time being, I didn't even have a calendar anymore.

My body was weak, uncoordinated, but the energy it took my brain to follow directions was significant, try and try again, even if was not done well. I wish I had videos of myself when I was younger, riding the bike and put it side-by-side of me riding the bike now. What you would see would be two very different people, but inside, I am the same person.

One thing that the hospital and community classes that I taught over the years and raising my own children have one thing in common, I didn't have to do everything alone. Others were there or nearby. Recovering from a stroke was no different. There was no way I could get better and regain what I did without everyone working together. If it was the helper's job, they did it without being asked twice. If it was family or friends, they did it because of love.

Do you know how you can tell the difference between a patient, a visitor, and a hospital employee? It depends whether they are lying in a bed, sitting by the bed, or they are standing and looking down at the person lying in the bed. Patients wear gowns; visitors wear whatever they want; employees wear a name tag. I have been all three.

It seemed like an odd time for me to become an expert on the brain, but I did learn parts of my brain and what it was responsible for. Each person who has a stroke or dementia is unique. Here's a simple example of the brain damage of these two conditions, at least in my situation: a stroke is a sudden loss of abilities and cognition, then slowly regaining some of the bodily functions; dementia is slowly losing abilities and cognition taking place over a period of time.

I am on the sixth year of sending out emails and texts with errors, typos, misspelling a person's name, forgetting something or someone. I can read and read a note over and over looking for mistakes and omissions, but you know what I am trying to say. I hope there are more thank you's in this story than mistakes.

"THANK YOU" ARE THE WORDS AND THE TIME TO SAY THEM IS NOW.

Thank you for joining me in my celebration of little steps. Ta Da!

Thanks for helping me and thanks for contributing to the possibility of a happy future for me.

Thanks for getting me to the next place and for taking a walk with me.

Thank you for reaching out to me and my family, the calls, notes, cards, emails, texts, visits, flowers, facebook posts, friendship, and good wishes. This includes good words spoken years ago; they may be the most valuable and powerful.

Thanks to all the Helpers, the Listeners, the Sharers, the Dreamers, the Hand Holders, and the Encouragers.

Thanks for giggles when everything was so serious.

Thanks for appearing magically at the exact right time.

Note. The Reason for lists. The lists are homage to the challenges I faced after the stroke of not being able to recall only a few items at a time.

Each and every one of you have been in my thoughts the past 6 years, reminding me who I was and that I could do whatever it took to get me here. I am sure we have had very serious conversations, but I remember laughing and feeling better. Your kindness and good thoughts has made all the difference. I have mentioned some of the people in this story who offered a helping hand that got me here today. Here are a few more lovely people and I am sorry that there are missing names.

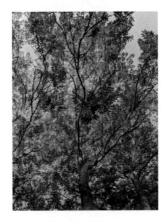

The manager and employees at Panera Bread in Plymouth kept me safe until the City of Plymouth Mi. Emergency Services, aka 911 arrived quickly.

St. Mary Mercy Hospital, Livonia, Mi. Everyone from the Emergency Room, in-house care recovery, and outpatient recovery. University of Michigan, Canton, Ann Arbor, and Livonia. My primary care physician, social worker, neurologist, urologist, physical therapists, and occupational therapists.

Illustrator: Ed Good, my brother, edgood11@gmail.com

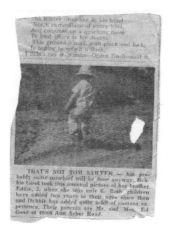

THAT'S NOT TOM SAWYER — but probably some mischief will be done anyway. Debbie Good took this unusual picture of her brother Eddie, 3, when she was only 6. Both children have added two years to their ages since then and Debbie has added quite a bit of camera experience. Their parents are Mr. and Mrs. Ed Good of 49000 Ann Arbor Road.

Editors and Readers

BookBaby

Dawn Ham-Kucharski

Brad Kadrich

Melissa Barnes

Marg Moxnes

Andrew and Justine MadonnaJohn Madonna and Rebecca Mitrovich

Mark Madonna and Amanda Xydis

Marcel Madonna

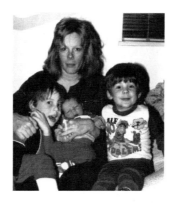

(Andrew, Mark, John, and Mom)

Aphasia Interpreter: Marcel Madonna

"How to Start and Finish a Book" Advisors

Joel Thurtell

Irene Elliot

Jennifer Adkins

Gerald VanDusen

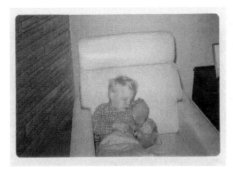
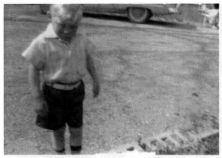

(Jeff Good. Permission to use granted by Jeff Good)

Jeff Good knows everything, especially about plants, flowers, and trees, just like CW. Thank goodness. Heidi remembers everything else. Thank goodness, too.

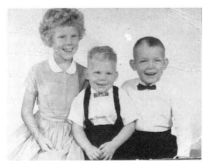
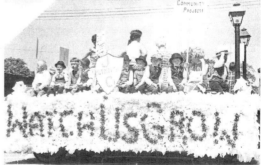

(Deb, Jeff, Ed. "Community Projects", Fourth of July Parade, Ed, Jeff, Deb)

Theresa Good, who is very kind, and all my dear Cousins, Aunts, Uncles, Nieces, Nephews, extra hugs for Jake Peters, and safe travels for Laura Nelson and Coddiwomple.

Lori Steward, how lucky we are, and Lynne Welty, thanks for watching over us.

Judy Shellhaas, John Shellhaas, Jason Shellhaas, Jess Vankoningsveld and Morgan Vankoningsveld, Mrs. Hirth, Harland and Dorothy Smith, Bernie Zeiler, and Marg Moxnes.

Colleen Riley Schroder was in Plymouth for the 50th Anniversary for the Class of 69, Plymouth High School a few years ago. Colleen asked me if, when we met all those years ago, did I think we would still be friends after fifty years. I answered, "Yes".

Mary, Mike, Maggie, and Matt Mitrovich, Randy Tesch, Frank and Loretta Keehl, David, Corkie, and Stephanie Lawton, Lucy Gavin, Jill Johnson, Barbra Wells. Sayre Fox, Melissa Barnes, Mary Novrocki, Sally Welch, Wyatt Hazlett, Jon Cassino, Rakesh and Sarita Sharma, Aarti, Stefan and Aaliyah Huber, Anjali Sharma, Jennifer, Gemma and Cameron Munson, Elizabeth, Hugh, and David Burley, Kim Delin, and Leis Dauzet-Miller.

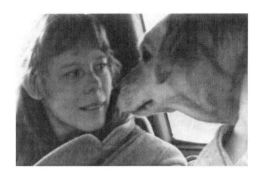

(Deb and sweet Freedom. Dave, Corkie, and Stephanie's dog, aka the much loved member of their family)

My music and baseball buddy, Jamie and the Jones and family. Louie Karras, Kathy Smalley and Alex Karras, Katie Hiltz, Rachel Koelzer,

Gabby McCall, Katelin Thomas Colvin, Jesse Jenkins, Jack Flynn, Mark LaPointe, Brian Paton, Jeff Powers Alex Ham-Kucharski, Dawn and Rich Ham-Kucharski, Sandy Sagear, Vonnie Bench and Tim Sagear and family, Jerry and Becky Trumpka, Dennis Jones, Scott Thomas, Sean Kahlil, Kurt Kuban, Steve Anderson, Dr. Anna Booher, Father Philip Schmitter, Stephanie and Brad Naberhaus, Building Bridges Therapy Center, and Lorraine and Donald Zaksek.

Dreamers: Rachelle Vartanian, Living and Learning Enrichment Center, Katie Howard, (who figures things out and listens to herself), Kristen Lamberson, (adventurer and traveler), Julie Giarratano, (who kept me company when the boys were being foolish), Kirbi Fagan and Nick Bair, (you are the only two people that I would like to go back in time with. Maybe we could be seven and go to summer camp. I think it would be cool.)

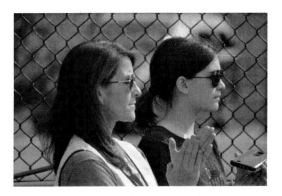

(Lisa Howard and Katie Howard supporting Miracle League of Plymouth players. They have supported me in countless ways, like so many others. Permission to use granted by Lisa and Katie Howard)

My neighbors, who tell me all the news in the neighborhood, keep an eye on me, and make me laugh: Baylin, Lukas, Jaxon. Kimmie and Dan Ervans, Becky and Ron Brodzik, Korey Brodzik, and Kyle Brodzik.

Nicole MacGregor, Emily Kaatz Cilibraise, Lisa Miller Harthun, Margaret Antio, Barbie Bouffard, Tricia Kennedy, Mike Howell, Lisa Howard, Gail and Mike Maloney, Jake Maloney, Lynne, Bob Hendzell and family, Lori and Craig Lee, Ruth and Larry Martin, Susan Lesser, Cindi Fry, Anya Linda Dely Dietz, Cathy Donaldson, Katie Donaldson, Melody Petrul, Nancy Oz, Deb Wardell, Michelle Dillon, Marisa Downs, Alicia Van Pelt, Kathy Koszegi, Lucy French, Lauren French, Tricia French, Susan Stoney, Patti VanDusen, Lauren Gohl, Kristen Smelser, Gayle Harshman, Nancy White, Teri Furr, Bernadette Glowski, Cheryl Fletcher Greening, Deborah Dooley, Karry Eckles Lancaster, and Amy Neale, Darrin Silvester, Kelly O'Donnell, Oliver Wolcott, Nick Moroz, Paul Sincock, and City of Plymouth Commissioners.

O.T. (Occupational Therapists) and M.T. (Massage Therapist), "Scraftie" classmates and Mrs. Horton. I took an anatomy class at Schoolcraft. After the first anatomy test, Mrs. Morgan told the class that everything we learned for the test, we needed to remember, even the Citric Acid Cycle. She was right. That was a good lesson to learn. To my fellow O.T. "Scrafties", the baby you gave me a baby shower for in our classroom, is 38 years old.

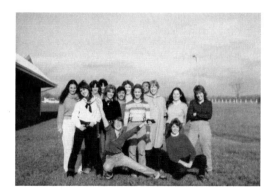

(OT Scrafties, Deb, Baby Andrew-to-be, Shower, in between classes)

I grew up and I live in the same town only a few feet from the houses I lived in. Those places I liked, but are gone, Cloverdale's, Daly's Restaurant, Kresge's, the Box Bar, Minerva's Dunning, P & A Theater. Happily, Bode's Restaurant is still open, Kemnitz Candy, the Plymouth Library, the Penn Theatre, PARC / Central Middle School / Plymouth High School, Starkweather School now condos. Thank you, Patricia and Mark Malcolm, Wendy Harless, and Don Soenen.

Still is in business. I am happy for that: Vanessa's Flowers have delivered many flowers to me at the hospital and my house. Graye's Greenhouse, new owner, Rachel Nisch and one of the gardeners, Jessica Anchor; It is a peaceful place, very therapeutic, and an important part of my entire life. Maggie & Me, a women's clothing store that has been in business since 1976. I love it. Whatever the occasion, I could find something to wear that was perfect. I never knew how important that would be in my recovery. Putting an outfit together was difficult at first. No worries. Maggie, Shelly and Alexandra know what I like and what I had at home that would go with the new clothes. That has been a luxury and therapeutic. I wish I had taken Flora and Blanche to the store. They would have loved it. I think of that often.

The Tuesday afternoon Plymouth Library Writing Group. Thanks for listening.

St. Peter's Lutheran Day School. My school and my teachers at St. Peter's School were: Miss Smart (Grades 1 – 3), Miss Ebe (Grades 4 – 5), Mr. Scharf (Grades 6 – 8), and Mrs. Goebel (Music Teacher for every grade). Miss Smart loved to teach children to read and she would suggest books that I may like and get lost in, The Boxcar Children, Cat in the Hat, and anything about foxes. Miss Ebe's hereafters taught me how to meditate and focus. And if I wasn't talking to my neighbor, I learned to love learning. Mr. Scharf read Edgar Allen Poe's stories to the class. Mrs. Goebel, well, she was the loveliest person in the whole world. I loved the Christmas Eve Pageant and all the practices we went to on Sundays in December. I wasn't a great singer, but I loved music, especially "Silent Night". Karen Stevens taught me to play the organ and never criticized me when she knew I didn't practice hardly at all, but I loved music. When St. Peter's celebrated their 50th anniversary, all my teachers were at the dinner. They weren't teaching at St. Peter's any longer. Can you imagine? All my teachers from First Grade through Eighth Grade in my old school.

Marg and Bern's parents: Dorothy and Harland Smith. Dorothy Smith was the leader of Girl Pioneers for quite a long time, as well as being involved in so many other things. Dorothy and Harland took us on many adventures. I remember Dorothy always had a lot of food at her house to be taken to some event. I remember eating the Pecans out of the Butter Pecan ice cream, I don't know which ice cream Marg was eating, but we took a little from every container. Bern is Marg's little sister, quite a few years younger than us. A few years ago we were all together, laughing, and having a very nice time in spite of us older girls being stinkers to her when she was just a little girl. Bern is now a fun grown up. We were reminiscing: we all remembered events differently, but it was fun. And now that we are all older, Bern will be driving us wherever we want to go.

I loved going to early church service; it was really early. We sat the front row. Harland, aka Smitty, was very cool. He was a powerful napper. In just a few minutes, he was dreaming and it didn't take very long for us to nod off, too. The Pastor knew that the sermon and the singing could get into our brains, eyes open or closed. Dorothy would poke the person next to hear and urge us all to open our eyes. Harland and Dorothy have always been the people I look up to. When Marg and I were in high school, Dorothy took us to see *"Dr. Zhivago"*. I went to the office and told them I was sick. The lady in the office said that she hoped I felt better soon. I did. I thanked her for her concern. Dorothy and Harland's house was the place that we "honorary daughters" spent as much time as we needed.

One of the gifts of going to this church and school was Pastor Berg's voice, the stained glass windows, and Bach. When I was little, after the church service, Rev. Hoenecke shook hands with everyone. He firmly held my hand, bent down, and spoke to me, still holding my hand. I have

167

included these people because one of the things that has been essential to my recovery was to have a brain full of memories of kind people who supported me, kept me safe, and shared the good in the world. "This is most certainly true." Rev. Edgar Hoenecke had beautiful white hair and he wore a navy blue suit.

As my friend, Amy Trombley, would ask at the end of each Allen Elementary School field trip. "Are we having fun yet?" Yes, Amy, I am having fun. How are you? I miss you.

My friend, Elaine Attridge drew a portrait of my grandson, Teddy, when he was 1 year old. When I was cleaning out a closet a few months ago, I discovered a portrait of my son, Mark when he was two years old. I didn't know Elaine then. I think we must have met her in Kellogg Park. Art is Elaine's way of showing the best in our world and that is a good thing.

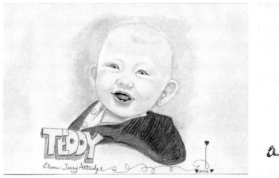 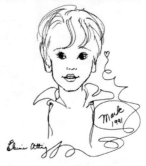

(Teddy and Mark)
(Permission to use granted by artist, Elaine Attridge, Andrew and Justine Madonna, Mark Madonna)

Special thanks to our house, sentimental treasures, and belongings. Extra special thank you to C.W., Flora, Bill, and Blanche for letting me follow you around.

I mentioned that when a baby is born at St. Mary Mercy Hospital, "Brahms Lullaby" is played on the overhead speakers throughout the hospital. Last year, during the pandemic, Lori Marie Key, a nurse at St. Mary Mercy Hospital, sang "Amazing Grace" to those on her floor, coworkers, and patients at a time there were no visitors allowed. A video went viral. "She (Lori) was invited to sing 'Amazing Grace' for the national audience at COVID-19 Memorial in Washington D.C. before President-elect Joe Biden and Vice President-elect Kamala Harris. The memorial was part of the inauguration events." (January 19, 2021. Detroit Free Press) "Amazing Grace" and "Brahms Lullaby". Lori Marie Key and Johannes Brahms. Music and Singing is the best medicine. It brought tears and hope to me. Thank you, Lori.

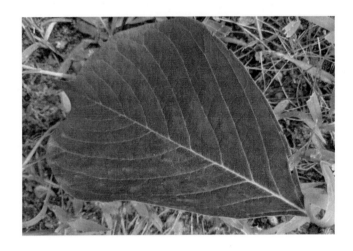

APPENDIX—
YEARS OF CELEBRATION

2021

Year 6, Month 6

2015: The Year of Stop, Drop, Survive. Roll. Rest. Recover. Thrive.

Mid 2015: The Year of Taking Care of Myself.

Late 2015: The Year of Taking it Easy.

2016: The Year of Playing Hooky.

2017: The Year of Playing Hooky continues.

2018: The Year of Being Happy.

2018: The Year of Wabi Sabi. *

2018: The Year of Ta Da. *

2019: The Year of No More Dragging my Right Foot.

2019: The Year of Strengthen my Core and Standing Tall.

2019: The Year of Looking Up, Not Down When I Walk, Stop Stooping,

2020 and Hereafter: The Years of Moving Through Life Vertical, with Grace and Ease.

2020 and Hereafter: The Years of Making Lists of all the things I love.

2020 and Hereafter: The Years of Kindness. Use Wisely. The Years of Time. Use Wisely.

2021 and Hereafter: The Years of Looking for fun and feeling groovy**

2021 and Hereafter: The Year of Rediscovering Culture and Opera.

Next Year: To Be Determined

   * Amy Krouse Rosenthal, *The Encyclopedia of an Ordinary Life*
   ** Paul Simon, *59ᵗʰ Street Bridge Song, Feeling Groovy*

DENNIS JONES
ON
SANDRA SAGEAR
WALL OF COURAGE

DENNIS Jones a licensed practicing local architect and artist designed and coordinated the Construction the Sagear Wall of Courage. He developed a dramatic presentation featuring an 18' x 9' multi-media design, which includes an alabaster sculpture and an extraordinary frame to display the names of all honorees.

Dennis M. Jones, February 27, 2002

"The image that moved me so regarding Sandra Sagear's life was picturing her as a small child strapped with leg braces and crutches. I imagined her constant struggle. Struggles that any healthy person would avoid or take for granted. Being a parent, I imagined the hardship her family must have endured. Yet Sandra, with the help of family and friends persevered and succeeded where others have failed. Such is the gift of the human spirit. It is with Sandra's spirit at heart that the Sagear Wall was conceived.

The Sagear Wall consists of several elements. Central to the design is a large, 430 lb. piece of white alabaster, carved in relief, depicting Sandra as an adult looking directly at herself as a small child. Sandra, the adult, appears to be reflecting on her life, whereas the child looks hopefully to the future. The white alabaster seems to capture Sandra's fragility and her calm, pure spirit.

The mural will measure approximately nineteen feet across and ten feet tall. Several outlined figures, carved into a wood panel, will grace the mural on both sides of the sculpture. The inclusion of these figures will suggest the support of family and friends or other students that have endured hardship and succeeded. A written biography of Sandra's life will be carved into the panel directly above the alabaster sculpture. The overall coloration of the mural will be white to compliment the alabaster sculpture and bring emphasis to Sandra's calm strength.

Other sculptural elements will include a child's crutch and leg braces. These two objects will be cast in lead and set upon a low wooden bench located on each side of the alabaster sculpture. The suggestion here recalls the manner in which Sandra may have removed and placed her crutches and braces at the end of her day. Lead was chosen as a material to suggest weight and burden. The lead will retain evidence of the casting process, the rough appearance further suggesting that these are objects of use with all the marks of their wear.

A frame made of lead is to also surround the entire mural. The names of past and future students that have endured hardships and succeeded will be engraved into the frame.

The completion of the Sagear Wall will bring me great pleasure to know that future generations will be encouraged to appreciate the hardship of others and their individual spirit to succeed."

SANDRA SAGEAR WALL OF COURAGE HONOREES AND SCHOLARS

Sandra Sagear Wall of Courage Honorees

The Sandra Sagear Wall of Courage is located at Plymouth High School, Canton, Mi.

Dennis Jones, local architect, artist and sculptor designed coordinated the construction of this wall. He developed a dramatic presentation featuring an 18' x 9' multi-media design, which includes an alabaster sculpture and an extraordinary frame to display the names of all honorees.

2007 Honoree:
Brian Geick

2004 Honorees:
Jeff Cardinal ~ David Foust
John Kreger ~ Scott Thomas

Sandra Sagear Scholars

2012
Allison Raylean ~ Bryan Ren
Caroline Wall

2011
Matthew Collingwood ~ Rachel Ferree
Shaniqwa Martin ~ Correy Rossi ` Elizabeth Rupp
Michelle Saucedo ~ Kristin Schultz
Davion Stackhouse ~ Mark Thompson

2010
Lauren Carnevale~ Kelly Hahn ~ Zachary Lizzio
Tabitha Mann ~ Anjali Patel ~ Melissa Pond

2009
Jessica Ayoub ~ Mohammad Bute
Chelsea Chadwick ~ Kirbi Fagan ~ Callie Gorlitz
Angelica Grady ~ Angelika Johnston
Vinny Lizzio ~ Ashley McKae ~ Alanna Mason
Brittany Robbins ~ Paul Zeuner

2008
Kathleen Balaze~ Alex Kemp ~ Felicia Matteucci
Leo McGhee ~ Arlesha McKinney ~ Megan Meek
Caitlin Quinn ~ David Smith

2007
Andrea Burdette ~ Angela Ayoub

2006
Leslie Baggs ~ Katlyn Harrison
Kathryn Huddleston ~ Kara McClure
Kathryn Morbitzer ~ Dave Mukerjee
Sara Schambers ~ Emily St. Onge
Kendra Summers ~ Alissa Vermeulen

2005
Kristine Clark ~ Sarah Letang
Sabrina Raben ~ Holly Ranta ~ Brad Zonca

2004
Brock Knowlton ~ Matt Tibaldi ~ Joseph Urban

2003
Amanda Bell ~ Corey Hensley
Kevin Kilgore ~ Sarah Palk ~ Matt Whalen

RESOURCES AND HELPERS

Primary Sources: what my husband told me, what friends and family told me, what my physician, therapists, and medical team told me, and the story my own medical records told.

No two strokes are the same. This story is not a medical document or meant to replace doctor or emergency services. If you suspect that you are not feeling well or that someone is in need of medical care, call 911. I am grateful that someone thought to call 911, even though I said I was "fine".

American Stroke Organization, www.stroke.org

Merriam – Webster Dictionary

The Plymouth Library & **MEL,** Michigan Electronic Library, and books on tape.

Jill Bolte Taylor, *My Stroke on Insight,* Doctor, Neuroanatomist, stroke survivor, author, TED Talk, *My Stroke on Insight.* Jill's stroke occurred on her left side. Her detailed observations of her stroke as it was occurring made quite an impression on me. (I had a left-sided hemorrhage.)

Oliver Sacks, *The Man Who Mistook His Wife for a Hat*

Steve Hartman, On the Road, CBS Sunday Morning, CBS Friday Evening News, and Kindness 101. Steve tells stories about people, all sorts of people in 3-minute videos and shares them with everybody; and then I can cry happy tears.

Valerie Eaton Griffith, *A Stroke in the Family,* 1970, Introduction by Patricia Neal

Diane Ackerman, *A Natural History of the Senses, Alchemy of Mind*

Andrea Olsen, *Body Stories*

Steve Parker, *The Body Atlas*

Paul E. Dennison and Gail Dennison, *Brain Gym*

Christopher Reeve, *Still Me, Nothing is Impossible: Reflections on a New Life*

Amy Krouse Rosenthal, *Encyclopedia of an Ordinary Life*, *Textbook*, *and I Wish You More*. I borrowed "Ta Da" from Amy and I use it all the time.

Erma Bombeck, *Motherhood, the Second Oldest Professions* and everything that Erma wrote.

Anna Quindlen, *Nanaville, A Short Guide to Happy Lives, Being Perfect*

Amy Tan, *Hundred Secret Senses and Where the Past Begins*

Kelly Corrigan, *Tell Me More, Lift*

Lesley Stahl, *Becoming Grandma*

Mary Oliver, *A Thousand Mornings*

Mitch Albom, *Tuesdays With Morrie*

Rachel Carson, *A Sense of Wonder*

Fred Rogers, *A Beautiful Day in the Neighborhood*

T. Berry Brazelton, *Touchpoints*

Vivian Gussein Paley

Jean Ayres, *Sensory Integration and the Child*

Viktor Frankl, Man's Search for Meaning

Gabby Gifford

Lou Gehrig

Franklin D. Roosevelt

Ruth Bader Ginsburg

Jimmy Carter

Jane Goodall

Dolly Parton

Elwood P. Dowd

The Beatles

Simon and Garfunkel, "Old Friends", "The Sound of Silence", and "The Bridge Over Troubled Waters". **Claire Wineland,** Claire's Place Foundation helps those living with cystic fibrosis.

https://clairesplacefoundation.org/

Emilia Clarke, aka Daenerys Targaryen, *Game of Thrones*, has had two brain hemorrhages and recoveries. She created "SameYou.Org".

https://www.sameyou.org/emilias-story

Patricia Neal, Academy Award winner had a brain hemorrhage in 1965. Her husband, **Roald Dahl**, is the author of *The BFG*. Read about Roald's contribution to Patricia's recovery.

How family tragedy turned Roald Dahl into a medical pioneer, Tom Solomon, The Guardian, September 12, 2019. https://www.theguardian.com/books/2016/ sep/12/roald-dahl-medical-*pioneer-stroke-hydrocephalus-measles-vaccination*

Joni Mitchell, polio survivor and recovers from a stroke, March 2015
Joni Mitchell still struggling to walk after 2015 aneurysm. Mark Savage, BBC News, October 27, 2020. https://www.bbc.com/news/ entertainment-arts-54703915
Joni Mitchell wrote the song "Woodstock", but she didn't go to Woodstock. *"Acts that almost made it to Woodstock",* Lauren Moraski, August 15, 2014, CBS News. https://www.cbsnews.com/pictures/acts-that-almost-made-it-to-woodstock/
Joni Mitchell's 'Blue' Album Turns 50, Ann Delisi, June 28, 2021, WDET, https:// wdet.org/posts/2021/06/28/91127-joni-mitchells-blue-album-turns-50/
I have a few things in common with **Joni Mitchell**. She didn't go to Woodstock; I didn't go to Woodstock. She wrote the song "Woodstock"; I love that song and so many more. Joni's album, "Blue", is 50 years old. I have been listening to it for 50 years. Joni had a stroke in 2015, so did I. Joni has fought the stroke and has improved a little at a time. Me, too.

In the words of **George Harrison,**

"Here comes the sun. And I say it's all right."

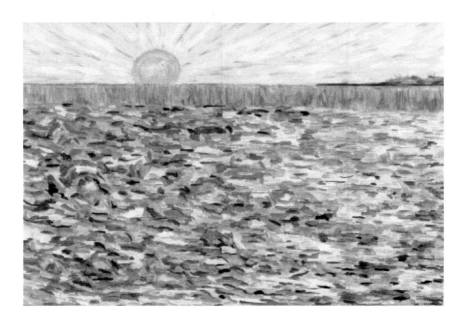

The Sun is Here

and

I'm home

(Permission to use granted by artist, Ed Good)

I survived that stroke. I started over. I recovered. I thrived ...

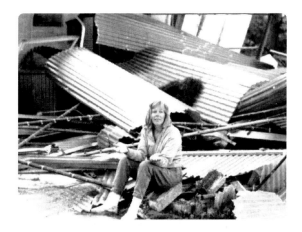

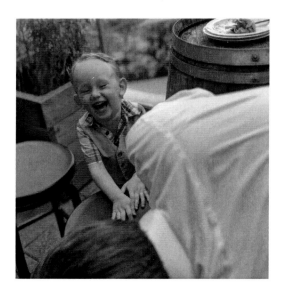

and we laughed.

(Permission to use granted by Andrew and Justine Madonna)